CONSTANCE MELLOR was born in Stoke-on-Trent. After she left school she became a full-time student at the Royal Academy of Music, studying singing and musical composition for three years. Her student years were followed by several years of public recitals and then by two and a half years of training to be a physiotherapist. After qualifying, she practised at various hospitals, and gradually built up a private practice in Hertfordshire where she has lived since 1934.

Since her retirement she has written one other book – *Handbook of Health* – and numerous articles for health magazines. Her philosophy of healing is strongly opposed to drug-therapy. Drugs treat only symptoms and not causes and the testing of drugs entails experimentation on dumb, defenceless creatures, causing them much pain and suffering.

D1635310

Natural Remedies for Common Ailments

Constance Mellor, M.C.S.P.

Mayflower

Granada Publishing Limited
Published in 1975 by Mayflower Books Ltd
Frogmore, St Albans, Herts AL2 2NF

First published in Great Britain by
C. W. Daniel Co. Ltd 1973
Copyright © Constance Mellor 1973

Made and printed in Great Britain by
Richard Clay (The Chaucer Press) Ltd
Bungay, Suffolk
Set in Monotype Times

This book is sold subject to the condition that it
shall not, by way of trade or otherwise, be lent,
re-sold, hired out or otherwise circulated
without the publisher's prior consent in any
form of binding or cover other than that in
which it is published and without a similar
condition including this condition being imposed
on the subsequent purchaser.
This book is published at a net price and is
supplied subject to the Publishers Association
Standard Conditions of Sale registered under the
Restrictive Trade Practices Act, 1956.

CONTENTS

INTRODUCTION

The first thing to know is a little about how your body works.

It is composed of millions of very tiny electrically-charged cells of various kinds (bone-cells, nerve-cells, blood-cells, gland-cells, brain-cells, etc.). The many differing kinds of cells are closely bonded together in differing groups, thus forming the many differing tissues, organs, and structures of the body. The number and type of cells in each group, and the manner in which they are bonded together, decides the resulting shape, size, and function of each different tissue, organ, or structure. For example, groups of bone-cells are grouped together in varying numbers and varying ways to form the many varying-shaped and varying-sized bones of the body. All cells are immersed in, and entirely surrounded by, intercellular fluid. This 'internal ocean' contains all the nutrients they need, as also the oxygen, to keep them alive.

The body's growth, repair-service, heat and energy production, are all dependent upon the proper nutrition of the 200 quintillion cells of which it is composed. If this is deficient, or if the intercellular spaces are clogged with waste-products so that oxygen cannot reach the cells and they cannot breathe properly, cell-function is impaired, resulting in symptoms of ill-health. Efficiency of the body's eliminative organs, which get rid of waste-products, is therefore very important, as is also a correct combining of foods. (See 'Compatible and Incompatible Foods'.)

The continuous changes taking place in every cell are known as cell-metabolism. This consists of a building-up of cell-structure known as 'anabolism', and a breaking-down of it, known as 'katabolism'. These chemical changes give rise to heat and energy.

Efficient cell-respiration and cell-metabolism depend not only upon an adequate supply to the cells of oxygen, of nutrients, and of water, but also upon an unhampered free circulation of the blood (the carrier of the oxygen, the nutrients, and the water.) This (a free unhampered circulation of the blood) depends very largely upon muscular exercise, without which it becomes sluggish and slow, with consequent impairment of cell-function. The rate of cell-respiration (i.e. the rate at which the cell extracts oxygen from the blood) is dependent upon the proper functioning of the body's endocrine glands, especially the Pituitary gland. If this gland produces too much or too little of its hormones, all the other glands are thrown off balance, cell-respiration is slowed, and cell-metabolism is seriously impaired, followed by ill-health in one form or another. However, glandular imbalance *can* be treated. Dr. Samuels treats it with short-wave (see *Appendix*).

Our body-cells are nourished by the food we eat, which is first broken up by the teeth, then churned up in the stomach, and broken down into simpler substances by digestive juices in the stomach and the intestines. Certain of these substances are then absorbed through the walls of the intestines into the surrounding blood-vessels, and carried away by the blood to all the tissues and organs of the body, each of which selects just those substances that it needs for the nourishment of the particular cells of which it is composed.

Some part of the cell-structure (the cell having done its building-up work) is then slowly burnt up, and for this burning-up process oxygen is needed, just as it is needed for all forms of combustion. Therefore oxygen, which is obtained from the air we breathe, must also be carried round in the bloodstream together with the food-nutrients. Like all other chemical reactions, the burning-up process (it is called oxidation) produces heat and energy, and it is this heat that keeps the blood and body warm. The need for breathing fresh oxygenated air at all times of the day and night, and of avoiding stuffy badly-ventilated rooms, is thus obvious, oxygen being *absolutely essential* for the process of oxidation with its resulting heat – and energy – production.

Water too is essential to the oxidation process. To maintain the blood's normal water requirement, it is necessary, in a temperate climate such as ours in Great Britain, to drink 1½–2 pints of water per day, in one form or another.

Water, as well as being essential to the oxidation process, is a solvent; it carries nutrients dissolved in it *to* the body-cells, and waste-products *from* the cells to the excretory organs. We lose water continuously (about 3½ pints daily), and to replace it is essential. It *is* replaced to the extent of about 1½ pints by the water-containing foods we eat (vegetables, salads, fruits, etc.) and the process of oxidation produces about a quarter of a pint. The remaining 1¾ pints required must be provided by drinking water – preferably distilled water, or natural Malvern water, or water in the form of fruit-juices, etc.

Ideally, all drinking water should be distilled water; it is the only sort of water that is a really suitable vehicle for conveying body-nourishment to the cells, because all other sorts – except natural spring-water such as Malvern water – are so dense.

All tapwater should be boiled before use, to remove the chlorine in it (this passes off in the steam); even cooking-water should be pre-boiled if the water in your district is hard and contains much calcium-bicarbonate, because hard water, when heated, coats food (as well as saucepans) with lime, and renders them indigestible. Natural spring-water (such as Malvern water) or distilled water, is of course the ideal sort to drink and to cook with; all are superior to tap-water, which nowadays is doctored with many chemicals. However, these chemicals (and all other impurities) can be removed by passing the water through a water-filter (made by Safari & Co. of 299 Ballards Lane, London, N.12). Malvern water is obtainable from most chemists, filters for filtering rainwater from Harrods of London.

Through countless ages, Man has developed and thrived

9

upon natural foods. Then, about 100 years ago, steel-roller mills, for grinding grain, replaced slower stone-grinding methods; white flour, deprived of its vital parts (its bran and its germ) was the resulting product. At about the same time, methods of sugar-refining were also developed, and sugar-consumption increased. It has gone on increasing ever since, so that now the average amount consumed by the majority of people – not only in hot drinks, but in jams, cakes, sweets, chocolates, etc. – is out of all proportion to bodily requirements. Furthermore, white sugar is over-refined and therefore an unbalanced food. It leaches vitamin B from other foods, because its own vitamins have been destroyed in the refining process. It is acid-forming, and a systemic poison. It should be replaced by natural sugars, such as those of honey, molasses, and dried fruits (especially dates). Honey is the purest form of sugar because it is untouched by Man.

Manufactured foodstuffs are mass-produced in factories and laboratories. They are, for the most part, foodless foods, of value only to the producers, who make big profits out of them. They are tinned, bottled, packeted rubbish, useless as proper nourishment for the body. Foods that are tampered with by Man – i.e. heat-treated, processed, tinned, bottled, or preserved – are killed stone-dead by the tampering, and certain it is that dead foods cannot put life into our bodies.

Our health – the health of the whole nation – has been taken out of our hands, and out of the hands of doctors, by the producers of these dead foods, as also by the manufacturers of chemical substances used *in* foods and *on* food-crops. These are the people – the makers of chemicals for use in and on foods, the food-technologists and the big-business men who employ them – who are responsible for present-day unnatural, over-refined, chemically-treated foods, and consequent widespread ill-health.

Unfortunately, ill-health cannot be cured by medical drugs, for the simple reason that these do not make good the nutritional deficiencies that cause it. Indeed, to a very great extent, corrective drugs actually *contribute* to ill-health and disease, by allowing the real cause of the trouble ('deficiency' foods, overcooked, and processed foods) to be overlooked.

Deficiency feeding gives initial warning signs and symptoms, such as stomach and bowel disorders, constipation, migraine, tiredness, nerviness, etc. These are suppressed if medical drugs are taken, so that their real cause is never treated, and gradually the sufferer's health gets worse, until eventually disease becomes established in his or her body.

It is not generally realized that the body can be over-fed yet under-nourished, and that imperfectly-nourished body-cells deteriorate and become diseased. Foods that are lacking in inorganic minerals and 'trace-elements' have no more building-power than have building-stones without a stone-mason, without whom they would never be built up into a structure. Similarly with food – *it is the inorganic-mineral content of the foods we eat that builds up their organic content into body-tissues.*

The low standard of feeding and of cooking in most big hospitals has been pointed out to the Ministry of Health by the Royal College of Physicians, and also by an eminent nutritionist Dr. Eddy.

What they reported to the Minister was confirmed by other reports from far and wide, and by a report from the Government, showing vitamin and mineral deficiencies in the food consumed by the patients. All this information has been completely disregarded by the Ministry, which has continued to regard adverse criticism of hospital-feeding and hospital cooking-methods as unjustified. Actually it is, of course, of tremendous importance, sick people being helped to recovery far more by properly-constituted, vitamin-and-mineral-rich food than by all the 'wonder' drugs in existence.

The past President of the Royal College of Physicians recently stated – 'Malnutrition in our hospitals is a very serious problem' – yet still nothing is done about it.

The National Health Service is costing the country more than fourteen hundred million pounds per year, a large part of which is spent on medicinal drugs for the treatment of ailments which are caused, basically, by nutritional deficiencies and errors. Surely it would be better spent on improving the standards of feeding and of cooking in hospitals, as also on health-education of the masses, most of whom have no idea of how to feed properly. It is, of course, up to doctors to teach their patients this. Unfortunately, doctors themselves know very little, if anything, about correct feeding, as they are trained to *treat* disease, not to *prevent* it, and the subject of Nutrition is not included in the curricula of medical-training schools.

Correct feeding and correct cooking-methods play a most important part in building up the sick body's recuperative powers – i.e. its ability to recover from illness. The foods that encourage a flow of nervous energy, and which therefore help recovery, are the sun-kissed green-leaf vegetables, salads, and fruits, all of which are full of vitality and life-giving energy. It is assumed that the sun gives them this vitality, though it is not understood exactly how it does it.

According to Dr. George Oshawa, author of *Philosophy of Oriental Medicine*, all disease is due to an imbalance of the sodium-potassium content of the blood. He advises sick people to live for 10 days on a 'mono-diet' of natural brown rice (cooked, of course), chewing each mouthful thirty times, and taking nothing to drink except MU tea. His dietetic beliefs are fully explained in a chapter headed The Macrobiotic Diet in Linda Clark's book *Get Well Naturally*.

Cooking is regarded by Dr. Hauschka, author of *Nutrition*, as a continuation of the vitalizing and ripening process of the sun's warmth. The correct way to cook vegetables, after washing and cutting them up, is to plunge them at once into a small amount of fast-boiling water, cover the pan with a tight-fitting lid, then allow them to cook gently till tender. (Potatoes should be cooked in their skins in a separate pan.) Slow gentle cooking extracts their juices and softens their tough outer fibres, making them easier to chew. Needless to say, the cooking-water should not be thrown away, because it contains the plant's valuable minerals. Cooking vegetables in pressure-cookers is not recommended.

Ideally, one's diet should consist of more raw than cooked foods, because raw foods have disease-preventing and therapeutic (healing) value, and are more easily and completely assimilated than cooked foods; so, anything that *can* be eaten raw, should be. All fats and all protein foods (with the exception of soya-beans, chick-peas, and lentils) are rendered indigestible and toxic by cooking; this means that cheese, milk, nuts, etc. should not be cooked, and that, if flesh- foods are eaten, they should be eaten in a semi-raw state (i.e. underdone). Egg-white should not be eaten raw, and, if it is eaten cooked, it produces toxic waste-products, so it should be discarded. Egg-yolk is best eaten raw or lightly cooked; its valuable lecithin, vitamins, etc. are thus conserved. Fats (animal *and* vegetable) should never be subjected to heat, because heat changes them chemically and renders them indigestible. This means that butter, margarine, cooking-fats, and oils should not be used for cooking, or incorporated in anything (such as bread, cakes, buns, pastry, etc.) that is cooked. Fats can, of course, be added to the cooked product. For example, cakes can be made without fat; then, when cooked, sliced and buttered.

Everyone should make it a rule to start every meal with something raw. There is a very important physiological reason for this, which is explained on page 203. The following foods should be avoided: All over-refined, chemically-treated, processed foods such as white flour, white sugar, white (pearl) barley, white rice, etc. (Brown barley and brown rice are available at health-foods shops); all factory-made foods, including factory-farmed meat, poultry, and battery eggs; all table-salt. If salt *is* used, it should be bio-chemic Bio-salt (Dr. Gilbert's) which is a balanced salt because it contains potassium and other minerals which balance the sodium-chloride in it. Refined table-salt is unbalanced because it is composed almost entirely of sodium-chloride. 'Herbamare' (a dried-vegetable salt) is a very good salt.

Introduction

A word of warning about drinking fluoridated water and about the use of aluminium cooking vessels. If you are unfortunate enough to live in a district where the water has sodium-fluoride added to it, step-up your daily intake of vitamin C. This will help to counteract the detrimental effect of the water on your health. In addition to foods rich in vitamin C (these are listed in my book *Handbook of Health*), eat several acerola or rose-hip tablets every day.

Aluminium cooking-vessels, kettles, etc. should be discarded (see *Why Aluminium Pans are Dangerous*, The C. W. Daniel Co., London) and replaced by good-quality enamel or stainless steel. Aluminium is a very soft metal, which is easily absorbed into the food or liquid cooked in it, and, in the long run, is slightly poisonous, as it cannot be completely eliminated by the body; it, therefore, tends to accumulate in the tissues, and is thought to be carcinogenic (cancer-causing). So, scrap all your aluminium ware; it is penny-wise and pound-foolish to keep it, as it will eventually lead to ill-health. A copper-bottomed stainless-steel kettle is the best sort to use.

Before going on to specific treatments, let us now examine the causes, prevention, and general treatment of disease.

It was the eminent physician and surgeon, Sir W. Arbuthnot Lane, who said: 'The chief cause of all disease is toxaemia, which means poison.'

Disease is an effort on the part of the body to throw off poisonous waste-matter and toxic substances, and although ailments may appear to be quite unalike, with differing symptoms, they invariably have (he believed) one basic cause, i.e. an unclean poisoned bloodstream.

Toxaemia is caused by a retention within the body of waste-matter and toxic substances, the cause of the retention being the fact that the eliminative organs cannot get rid of them as quickly as they are produced, and so they accumulate – chiefly in the large bowel – setting up putrefaction (a going-rotten process), with its putrefactive gases which poison the bloodstream.

14

All the waste-products of the body are the end-products of digestion. Most raw foods are completely digested, leaving very little waste-matter. All *cooked* protein foods, especially flesh foods, are robbed by cooking of their vitamins and digestive enzymes, thus preventing them from being completely digested. This means that they produce more waste-matter than raw foods, and it is of the kind that quickly putrefies in the large bowel, thus causing toxaemia. A contributory factor to toxaemia are the added substances ingested with the foods we eat and the water we drink, both of which are chemically treated nowadays. Toxins are also ingested with the fume-laden air we breathe. Deficiency foods, too, contribute to toxaemia, because they not only fail to provide the body with what it needs (i.e. with cell-nutrients), but clog it with what it does *not* need.

Mental and emotional disturbances, causing an imbalance of the vital electric-field within which cell-metabolism takes place, also produce toxins. When the soil of this electric-field is undisturbed by mental or emotional conflict, disease germs can (and do) live in it, but they cannot multiply or produce toxins, and so they remain quiescent and harmless to the body. It is only when the soil of the electric-field is disturbed, or when the blood is polluted with toxic wastes, that germs can develop and multiply, and become harmful. Thus it can be truly said that germs are not the *cause* of disease, but are merely a concomitant of it – a result, not a cause – and that *it is maladjustment of the body to mental and emotional disturbances, as well as deficiency foods and inefficient elimination of waste-products, that are the three main causes of disease*. To some extent, therefore, we cause our own disease, and control of it lies within the Psyche (the temperament) of the sufferer.

Other factors in the resistance of the body to disease are:

(*a*) The behaviour and condition of our etheric and spiritual bodies.

(*b*) The condition of our nervous system.

(*c*) The influence of the planetary bodies (chiefly the sun and moon).

But these are factors with which this book does not deal. It deals simply with two big causes of disease, i.e. with toxaemia, and with 'deficiency' feeding, and explains how to remedy them. (For information about the factors mentioned above, see *Some Unrecognized Factors in Medicine*, The Theosophical Publishing House, London.)

The chief aim in the treatment of any illness should be to build up strength and resistance by means of correct feeding, but it is useless to attempt to do this until the body has been thoroughly cleansed. Body cleansing is best achieved by rest, including rest from solid food for a day or two, plus cleansing washes (external *and* internal, if necessary). A preliminary bowel purge is also necessary sometimes.

Incomplete elimination of waste-products and of toxins from the body, due to inefficiency of the eliminative organs (the bowels, the kidneys, and the skin), causes retention of them in the body and a consequent poisoning of the bloodstream. This inefficiency of the eliminative organs is partly due to 'deficiency' feeding, partly to a lack of nervous energy. (Such a lack of nervous energy is known as Enervation.)

Deficiency feeding can be remedied (see my book *Handbook of Health*). The question is – what is the cause of Enervation, and how can *it* be remedied?

There are many causes of Enervation; the following are the commonest: the stresses and strains of life; excesses of all kinds, including excessive eating or drinking, excessive smoking, excessive indulgence; strains of all kinds (physical, mental, and emotional), including the strain of overwork or overplay; the strain of having to make important decisions and of having to cope with difficult situations and/or difficult people; the strain of having to live with difficult or uncongenial people, and of having to adapt to all sorts and conditions of people and of surroundings, including changeable climatic conditions. The above are but a few of the many causes of Enervation, leading to inefficiency of the eliminative organs, with consequent toxaemia, ill-health, and disease.

Symptoms of an acute illness (which usually has a name ending in 'itis', such as bronchitis, tonsilitis, appendicitis, colitis, etc.) are the outward signs that the body is trying to cleanse itself and to normalize its blood-condition. The body's instinctive intelligence, which is distinct and different from the intelligence of the mind, tells it to make the effort to cleanse itself when the accumulations of toxic substances and waste-products in the bloodstream become more than can be got rid of by the eliminative organs. Acute illness should, therefore, be regarded as a remedial and beneficial outlet, rather than as something to be feared and suppressed; for, if the body were too weak to make the effort to cleanse tself, it would simply die – of toxaemia. Moreover, if the symptoms of an acute illness are repeatedly suppressed (with medicinal drugs), the illness will become chronic, and chronic illnesses are much more difficult to cure than acute ones.

Given the right foods and the right environment, the body is a self-regulating, self-healing organism, capable of putting right its own troubles, though sometimes it can be helped in its efforts to do so by biochemic, herbal, and homoeopathic remedies. (More about these later.) The fight against disease really all depends upon the Life-force within the body.

If the inherent Life-force can be raised sufficiently, all disease is curable. How best to raise it is therefore the important question. The answer is – by conserving it, and the best way of conserving it is by REST. This may include a rest from solid food for a day or two, because the digestion of solid food uses up vitality. A light diet – or sometimes a diet of liquids only – is therefore advised in illness, chiefly because such a diet conserves vitality, but also because it gives the digestive organs a rest, and provides an opportunity for the intercellular spaces to get rid of accumulated debris. This debris, unless removed, clogs the spaces and prevents oxygen from reaching the cells, thus interfering with cell-respiration, cell-metabolism, and cell-efficiency.

Symptoms are outward signs of internal disorder; they are the means whereby the body draws attention to itself and asks for help. If they are very painful or unpleasant, they can be eased with natural remedies, but they should be studied, and their underlying cause ascertained, then treated. (This statement does not apply to accidents, only the symptoms of which *can* be treated, the cause of the symptoms being already known.)

Orthodox medical treatment of disease, with its symptom-suppressing drugs, vaccines, etc. usually only hinders the self-healing efforts of the body and makes recovery more difficult. (Again, this statement does not apply to accidents, because accidents are not diseases.) For example, if the symptoms that have been troubling you cease when your doctor gives you one of the many modern drugs (most of which are substances foreign to the body), it is not likely to be because the drug has cured the trouble; it is really because the body has had to switch its attention from its self-healing efforts (i.e. from its efforts to draw attention to itself) to an effort to get rid of the foreign substance (the drug) which is unacceptable to it.

According to the late Sir William Osler (an eminent physician and surgeon), when drugs are used the patient has to recover twice – once from the illness, and once from the drug.

Research scientists are working feverishly to produce new drugs to fight new strains of microbes in the human system. These new strains are resistant to drugs that have been in use for some length of time; therefore new drugs have to be found to fight them. Drugs are not the answer to disease-strains, either in man or plants. A pure bloodstream is the answer.

Drugs cannot cure diseases; disease continues. It is only its pattern that changes. Of course, just a few drugs *are* useful. These can, and do, give relief from pain and discomfort; for example, after an accident, as also during the terminal stages of a long and hopeless illness, when all one can hope to do for the sufferer is to give him (or her) some relief from pain and distress. Other drugs, as they do not treat the underlying *cause* of the symptoms, are at best purely palliative, and at worst an encumbrance to the body. The great danger of drug-therapy is that it masks the early signs (symptoms) of disease, which, if observed and studied, could be traced to their cause, and treated by natural means – i.e. by rest, by fasting and correct feeding, and by suitable herbal, homoeopathic, and biochemic remedies. Surgery should seldom become necessary.

The importance of the role of correct feeding in the prevention and treatment of ill-health and disease cannot be overestimated. Yet the vast majority of orthodox medical men and women pay little or no attention to it, probably because they receive little or no tuition in the subject at their medical-training schools.

It is not an exaggeration to state that, so long as cell-nutrition and cell-respiration is adequate, the body is practically proof against attack by disease-germs, there being no opportunity for them to gain a foothold and start disease-breeding activities in a properly-nourished body with a clean bloodstream and a normal mental and emotional life.

The quality of the soil in which our foods are grown is also of vital importance to the maintenance of health and the prevention of disease. Many eminent men of science, including Dr. Henry Gilbert, author of *Science, Sickness, and the Soil*; André Voisin, author of *Soil, Grass and Cancer*; Professor Schuphan, author of *Nutrition Value in Crops*; and Sir Albert Howard, author of *The Soil and Health* and many other books – all these eminent men (and many others) attribute a lack of vital substances in our foods to a lack of them in the soil in which the foods are grown – as well as to food-processing and food-refining. 'Put right the soil-deficiencies', they say, 'and this will put right the health of the animals and of the people who eat the produce of the soil.'

Introduction

The soil, from which plants derive their sustenance, should contain all the nutrients essential for building strong healthy cells and for strengthening the defence-mechanism of the plant. If any of these essential nutrient-minerals are lacking in the soil, the health of the plant, and its resistance to disease, suffers – just as the health and the resistance to disease of the human body suffers if any of them are lacking in the body's bloodstream (through lack of them in the foods eaten). A weakened defence-mechanism means that disease-organisms are able to gain entry into the body more easily. In other words, a lack of essential nutrients in the soil will result in a lack of them in the produce of the soil and in the animals and the people who eat the produce. Thus we get sick plants, sick animals, and sick people. *HEALTH, THEN, BEGINS IN THE SOIL.*

Surely, instead of working feverishly to produce new drugs to combat disease, it would be wiser for research scientists to put the horse before the cart (instead of the other way round) and to concentrate on studying how best to build up the health of the soil. Plants, and the animals and people who eat them, would then become so healthy that they would not need drugs to fight disease-germs.

Soil Science, which seeks to heal the soil, so as not to have to heal the animal or the man, is therefore the basis of *Preventive Medicine, the Medicine of Tomorrow*. But, except for the Soil Association, and the Henry Doubleday Research Association, present-day Science concentrates on 'results', not on 'causes' – on the production of drugs to deal with ill-health that is basically due to 'deficiency' foods grown in 'deficiency' soil. To cite an example, a deficiency of trace-elements in the soil, caused by prolonged use of large quantities of nitrogenous fertilizers, seriously endangers the health of the animals and of the humans who eat the produce of the soil. Such fertilizers upset the balance of the mineral-elements in the soil, and this has the effect of upsetting the balance of the mineral-elements in the blood of the humans who consume its produce. For example, an imbalance in the ratio of magnesium to potassium in the blood, due to an imbalance of these minerals in the foods eaten, aids the development of cancer, and of thrombosis. Such an imbalance in the foods we eat *can*, of course, be due to food-processing and food-refining, as well as to an imbalance of the soil-minerals. For instance, white bread (and other things made of white flour) is a deficiency food, in which the ratio of magnesium to potassium is unbalanced because it is made from grain that has had its husk and its germ removed in the milling. The grain itself may have been grown in mineral-rich soil, whose mineral balance had *not* been upset by artificial fertilizers. In this case, therefore, the mineral-imbalance of the flour is produced by its refining, which has removed the mineral-rich germ and husk.

Beware, therefore, of 'deficiency' foods, and make doubly sure of avoiding them by buying wholewheat flour (and bread) from a health-foods shop, and by growing your own crops (as far as possible), fertilizing the soil with home-made compost, and with dried seaweed mixed with Humin C. (from the Compost Research Centre, Grantham, Lincs. – See also F. C. King's *The Compost Gardener*, Faber and Faber).

Some American doctor-nutritionists, who are more food-conscious than British doctors, believe that most diseases are due not only to eating over-refined 'deficiency' foods, grown in 'deficiency' soil, but also to eating incompatible foods together at the same meal. This faulty habit causes fermentation in the stomach, and produces toxic gases in the large intestine. Constipation, and all digestive disturbances resulting from it, such as duodenal ulcer, colitis, appendicitis, diverticulitis, gall-stones, liver disfunction, etc. are due, they say to eating 'deficiency' foods *and* to faulty food-combining. (See *Superior Nutrition*, *Health Via Food*, and *Food Combining Made Easy*, in 'Books for Further Reading'.)

Their advice, as far as it goes, is sound, stressing (as it does) the importance of not mixing up a whole conglomeration of different classes of foods in the stomach at one and the same meal, and of eating just *one* kind of 'complete' protein at a meal. (If several kinds are eaten, it only makes extra work for the liver and other digestive organs, and contributes no extra benefit.) But what they have omitted to say is that about half of one's total daily intake of 'complete' protein should be eaten together with some carbohydrate (i.e. with food of a starchy nature) – otherwise, the protein is useless for body-building. The liver, by means of potent ferments, makes it useless by eliminating the nitrogen from the amino-acids of which it is composed. But if it is accompanied by glucose (derived from the carbohydrate food of the meal), the activity of the liver-ferments is stopped, and the amino-acids retain their nitrogen, which can then be used for body-building.

The vast majority of our British doctors seem ignorant of the close relationship that exists between soil, food, and health, their medical training having stressed the curative aspect of medicine rather than the preventive aspect. Almost the only form of preventive medicine that *is* practised by them is vaccination against smallpox, and inoculation against whooping-cough, diphtheria, poliomyelitis, etc. This form of disease-prevention is very hazardous, and may do more harm than good; moreover, its power of prevention has not been proved; its power to do harm *has*. It should be more widely publicized that the causal germs of such diseases cannot live and multiply in a clean and healthy bloodstream, which is therefore the best and safest kind of insurance against attack by them – indeed, against attack by all disease.

Wise parents do not have their children vaccinated against smallpox, or inoculated against measles, whooping-cough, or polio. Vaccination is not a 'health' measure; indeed, it is an unhealthy measure, with risk of permanent damage to health. (See *The Hazards of Immunisation* by Sir Graham Wilson, M.D., Athlone Press; also *The Blood-poisoners* by Lionel Dole, Gateway Book Co., also free leaflets published by the Anti-Vaccination League, 2a Lebanon Road, Croydon, Surrey.)

The greatest single factor in the retaining (*and* regaining) of health is correct feeding. This ensures efficient elimination of waste-products via the bowels and kidneys – thus a clean bloodstream – and this is proof against germs and viruses, which can live and thrive *only* on waste-products and in unclean surroundings. Medicines are of little help if the nutrition of the body is incorrect or inadequate.

When first doctoring and medicine was studied and practised, some hundreds of years ago (chiefly by scholarly men, who used only herbal remedies), more importance was attached to the *prevention* of disease than to its treatment, and the then-doctors concentrated on the teaching of Nature's laws, and on the use of Nature's remedies. They understood the value of fasting – not only for spiritual reasons (as self-discipline), but for health reasons. They were doctors in the real sense of the word; (the word doctor means teacher). Unlike present-day doctors who seem bent upon pushing as many things as possible *into* the patient, they aimed at trying to remove noxious substances *out* of the patient, and they prescribed very little in the way of medicine to be taken *into* the body. In addition to fasting, they used also the following eliminative methods of treatment:

Blood-letting (*Venesection*). This was used for high blood-pressure, over-thickness of the blood, too much blood, coronary congestion, thrombosis, embolism, fracture of the skull, shock (to prevent the formation of blood-clots), post-operative embolism (to prevent *and* cure), drowning, strangulation, chest-wounds, meningitis, and pneumonia.

Purging. This was used for most common ailments, and for purification of the blood and of the bowels, as also for obesity. The purge used was usually aloes (a herb).

Sweating. This was used for elimination of poisons through the skin (and still is). It was usually combined with Hydrotherapy (water-treatments).

Blistering. This was used for all forms of rheumatic ailments, including arthritis. It was also used for angina pectoris, and other forms of heart trouble, the idea being to draw the gouty deposits and other noxious substances in the heart muscle to the surface of the body, thus assisting their elimination from the body via the skin.

Cupping. This was used to assist the expulsion of inflammatory products in the skeletal muscles, e.g. for lumbago. It was also used for heart pain, chronic bronchitis, and other chest troubles. Nowadays, it is used for Disseminated Sclerosis. (See chapter on 'Cupping' in *Some Unusual Methods of Healing* by Leslie Korth, D.O., Health Science Press.)

Vomiting. This was occasionally employed for intractable chest complaints such as chronic bronchitis, bronchial asthma, emphysema, etc. It was also often used for mental patients, because it was believed that vomiting had the sobering effect of 'bringing down to earth' certain types of mentally-deranged people.

Fasting is a rational and scientific way of cleansing the body and of ridding it of disease-poisons. It is sometimes confused with starving, which is something quite different. Starving is going without food when the body is needing it and suffering for lack of it; fasting is deliberate refraining from food when the body is in such a toxic state that food cannot be properly digested and assimilated, and when the body is therefore better able to rid itself of toxins by refraining from food.

Everyone should make a habit of fasting occasionally (at least once a month) for twenty-four hours, irrespective of whether or not he or she is well or not. It is a precautionary measure which allows the overworked organs of elimination to 'catch up' and to avoid getting behindhand with their important work. It also gives the digestive organs a bit of well-deserved rest. During the twenty-four hours, only liquids should be ingested, chiefly freshly-pressed vegetable or fruit juices.

Once a year (more often if you eat flesh foods), the fast should last two or three days, and should be followed by two weeks on a cleansing (chiefly raw-food) diet, consisting of fresh ripe fruit, sun-dried fruits, raw vegetable-juices, cooked vegetables, and salads – a diet that excludes all protein foods, fats, starches, and sugars. The best time to choose for this yearly 'spring-clean' is mid-summer, when it is warm, when fresh fruits and salads are at their best and most plentiful, and when this bodily 'spring-clean' can be combined with outdoor exercise, with sun and air baths, and with relaxation of body and of mind. It will then do you the maximum amount of good, and will set you up in health for the coming year.

During the preliminary 2–3 day fast, only fresh-fruit juices, raw vegetable juices, drinks of Malvern water and cups of herb tea (such as English herb-tea or Potter's alpine-herb tea), should be ingested – no solid food whatsoever. Lemon-juice (or milk) and a little honey may be added to the tea.

It is advisable to start the first day of fasting with a heaped teaspoonful of Epsom salts in $\frac{1}{2}$ pint of hot water, followed by a drink of hot tea. If this does not thoroughly purge the bowels, take two doses next morning (separated by 20–30 minutes) and a 1 pint warm-water enema at bedtime. It is essential that the bowels should be given a thorough cleansing, but this Epsom salts purge should be used only whilst fasting, to assist the cleansing action of the fast.

Epsom salts (magnesium sulphate) has a strong attraction for carbon, so, when a strong dose of salts is taken, what happens is this: the massive dose of salts saturates the entire lining of the digestive tract, and by a process of osmosis, attracts (and thus removes) the carbonaceous wastes out of the blood as it circulates around the external surface of the digestive tract, these carbonaceous wastes being drawn *out of* the bloodstream (by the attractive power of the salts) *into* the digestive tract. Here they pass on, until they eventually reach the eliminative organs which expel them from the body. Thus, all parts of the digestive tract and of the trunk are cleared of pent-up accumulations of waste-products and impurities. Such accumulations clog the intercellular spaces, preventing proper cell-respiration and cell-nutrition; for neither oxygen nor nutriment can reach the cells if the spaces round them are clogged.

Elimination of waste-products and impurities via the skin can be helped by taking, once or twice a week, a hot bath in which about a pound of common Epsom salts is dissolved. No soap should be used, but the body should be frictioned all over with a brush. (A man's nylon hair-brush is suggested.) Finish with a cool shower, if possible, then dry with a rough towel till the skin is red and glowing. (People with heart trouble should not have the water too hot.) A clean cotton vest should be worn next to the skin, and should be changed three or four times a week; so, too, should socks and stockings.

Now a few words about the general treatment of illness, before going on to the treatment of specific ailments. In illness, it is never only one particular organ or tissue that is affected; it is the entire body. Its powers of self-healing can be mobilized and assisted by one (or more) of the following therapies: Fasting, dieting, hydrotherapy (external and internal), homoeopathic, herbal, and biochemic remedies, sleep therapy, etc. In the initial stages, most acute illnesses should be treated on the lines laid down for 'Fevers'. (For details of 'Pyonex' treatment, Acupuncture, etc. see *Some Unusual Methods of Healing* by Leslie Korth, D.O., Health Science Press.)

Biochemic remedies are composed of the inorganic minerals required by our body-cells. Under normal conditions of health, the body-cells obtain these essential inorganic minerals from the nourishment (the organic food-substances) brought to them by the bloodstream, and they are able to utilize them. These inorganic minerals are the work-men who build the structure of the cell; without them, food would be as useless as a pile of bricks without a brick-layer. But, in illness, the body-cells are so weakened that they are often unable to take up and to utilize the rather coarse-grained inorganic minerals in the nutrients brought to them, and the consequent lack of one (or more) of these vital minerals means that the cells starve (i.e. are not built up), deteriorate, and die. The minerals composing the biochemic remedies are very finely-ground, and are therefore more easily absorbed than those in the food-nutrients; the sick cells are thus able to absorb them, and to recover their ability to function normally. The biochemic doctor's clue as to which of the twelve basic minerals to prescribe is given by the nature of the patient's symptoms. (For further reading on the subject, see the Introduction to Dr. Geo. Carey's book *The Biochemic System of Medicine*, published in Calcutta, but obtainable from a Free Library.)

The method of taking the remedies is important; they should be allowed to dissolve slowly under the tongue, *not* swallowed with a drink, like most other remedies. This is because, if they are swallowed, their constituent minerals will get mixed up with the stomach-acids, which will change them chemically, so that they will reach the cells in a changed state; whereas if they are allowed to dissolve under the tongue (thus by-passing the stomach) they will remain unchanged chemically and will be absorbed direct into the bloodstream via the walls of the mouth, the throat, and the tiny blood-vessels therein, thus reaching the body-cells in a chemically-unchanged state. Homoeopathic remedies should also be taken in this way. (See 'Homoeopathy' page 218.) Herbal remedies are generally taken in the form of a tea, by pouring boiling water over the herb in a teapot, and allowing it to infuse for a short time. Some herbal-tea recipes are given on page 198.

Fear should not be allowed to paralyse the electro-magnetic forces of the body when it is sick. Fear intensifies disease-conditions, and inhibits the power of the body's healing forces. So try to keep a serene mind, with faith in your body's recuperative powers.

In *The Practice of Nature-Cure*, (Gateway Book Co., Croydon, Surrey) Dr. Lindlahr says:

> The positive mind and will are, to the body, what the magneto is to the automobile. As the electric sparks from the magneto ignite the gas, thus generating the power that drives the machine, so the positive vibrations generated by a confident and determined will, will create in the body the positive electro-magnetic currents which incite and stimulate all vital activity. Therefore the victory in acute diseases is conditioned by absolute faith, confidence, and serenity of mind on the part of the patient. Do not convey alarm to the millions of little cells doing battle in the inflamed parts; speak to them like a commander addressing his troops. Say to them 'We understand the laws of disease and cure; we know that these febrile and inflammatory symptoms are the result of Nature's healing efforts; we have perfect confidence in Her wisdom and in the efficiency of Her healing forces. This fever is merely a good house-cleaning, a healing crisis; we are eliminating morbid matter and poisons which were endangering life and health.'

In *A New Health Era* (George Harrap) Dr. W. H. Hay says:

> There is no treatment under the sun that can add one atom of resistance to any organ, for resistance is determined by our manner of living. And, just as surely as medicine cannot make hair grow or replace a finger-nail, so just as surely can medicine do nothing constructive for any disease. It can change the symptoms, relieve pain, cause the bowels to move with the whip of laxatives, and it may delude us into thinking that our condition is better after a remedy than before; but in any way to change the con-

dition of the body for the better is not within the powers of therapeutics. *Nature* creates, maintains, and regulates the organs of the body, and Nature alone can do this.

Only when humanity has become wise enough to understand the origin of its own illness, and sane enough to correct these origins, will the physician become the teacher and the watch-dog of health, instead of the tinkerer with end-results, which is what he is at present.

Dr. Hay goes on to say that it is foolish and unkind to try and persuade the sick person to eat when he or she has no desire for food – that the kindest thing we can do is to omit all mention of food until the patient expresses a desire for something to eat. He says: 'Many a case of acute illness has been brought back to safety by the use of simply natural juices, with solid food of every sort omitted until recovery was well on the way and the patient again expressed a desire for food.'

There are certain natural laws that govern all life. The fact that our civilized, social, and economic systems make it well-nigh impossible for us to conform to these natural laws does not in any way prevent or alter their inexorable operation. Civilized man, through not obeying these laws, must pay the price of disobedience, the price being ill-health. Nature cannot be fooled nor cheated, and Man reaps always what he sows.

Only by a return to natural living based upon natural laws, and to natural (mostly uncooked) foods, is it possible for civilized man to experience the full health and happiness to which he is heir, and to command them as a right. Any foods that cannot be eaten raw (such as flesh foods) should not be eaten at all.

It may not be possible for us to eat *only* uncooked foods, but it is possible for us to omit cooked protein foods from our diet, and to eat fruits and vegetables in their raw state. *Unfired food is best, because it retains its vitamins and enzymes intact. Cooking kills them.*

Cooking also speeds up the oxidation of foods (their propensity to combine with oxygen in the air) and, once foods have been oxidized, they cannot be re-oxidized in the body, and therefore are no longer of any real value as body nourishment, though such a loss in value may not result in ill-health until middle-age or even later. Foods combine with oxygen in the air less readily if the air is cold than if it is warm (room-temperature); hence the desirability of keeping foods in a refrigerator or in air-tight containers in a cold place, so that oxygen cannot combine with them.

The stress and strain of present-day life, the rush and hurry of it, the endless difficulties of earning one's living in the face of fierce competition in the human rat-race, very often having to do so in the smoke and fume-laden air of towns and cities – all these adversities are the outcome of civilization (so-called), and are highly unnatural, ill-health and disease being the inevitable result.

This book, and the books mentioned in it, will be, it is hoped, a help to thousands of sick people at present suffering under the well-meaning but unhelpful efforts of doctors to cure their ailments. Many of these people have gone from doctor to doctor, in the hope of being cured, only to find that, instead of getting better, they are getting worse; indeed, in many instances they have been pronounced incurable – doomed to a death-in-life existence.

The true art of healing consists in *aiding* Nature, not in thwarting Her by giving suppressive drugs, vaccines, etc. Given the right tools, Nature (our subconsciousness) can do the job of healing, for healing is Her own prerogative, which cannot be delegated to doctors. Nature does the healing, though the doctor usually gets the credit for it!

ACCIDENTS AND FIRST AID
IN THE HOME

A first-aid box should be kept handy in every home. In addition to cotton-wool, gauze, lint, bandages and adhesive plaster, it should contain homoeopathic Calendula tincture, Arnica, and Urtica Urens.

CALENDULA TINCTURE. This is used for cuts, wounds, bites, stings, burns in the mouth from over-hot food, as a mouthwash after tooth extraction, and for varicose ulcers (and other parts that will not heal). First make a lotion, using 20 drops of the mother-tincture to a teacupful of boiled water that has cooled. Then, for wounds, divide this lotion into two small bowls (previously scalded). Use one for bathing the wound, using a piece of cotton-wool, working from the centre outwards. In the other bowl, soak a piece of sterile gauze large enough to cover the wound, and also a piece of lint. When the wound is cleaned, place the gauze then the lint, over it. Cover with cotton-wool or clean flannel, and bandage firmly but not too tightly.

If the wound oozes pus, the gauze will stick and will have to be gently removed after an hour or two by sopping it with warm water, to loosen it. A clean piece, soaked as before in the lotion, should be applied and covered, as before, with a clean piece of lint soaked in the lotion. If the wound does not ooze pus, the gauze need not be renewed, but the lint should be resoaked in the lotion and replaced over the gauze, every 3–4 hours.

A 3,000-year-old Chinese remedy for suppurating wounds is bread-mould; the modern equivalent is penicillin.

An animal's remedy is its own saliva, and we should not fear to use our own saliva for wounds, bites, stings, etc., as saliva is antiseptic and healing, and can safely be used if no other remedy is handy.

If the patient is suffering from shock or is in pain, precede all treatment with a dose (2 pilules) of homoeopathic *arnica 12x.*, every hour (or oftener) until the pain eases. Another excellent remedy for pain and shock is Dr. Bach's rock-rose 'rescue' remedy. (The dose is 3–4 drops in water.) See page 210.

ARNICA TINCTURE. This is used for bathing bruises, blows, and sprains, if the skin is unbroken. If broken, Calendula lotion (marigold) should be used.

URTICA URENS. For burns and scalds, follow the instructions given above for wounds, using tincture of Urtica Urens Ix. (10 drops to half a cupful of boiled water). But for burns caused by acids, use *Bicarbonate of Soda* (1 teaspoonful to ½ pint of boiled water). Quickly soak a pad of lint or gauze in the lotion and apply it speedily, the idea being to exclude the air from the injured part as quickly as possible. Cover the pad with a thick piece of cotton-wool and then with a piece of oiled silk and a bandage. Moisten the pad with the lotion every hour or so. If the burn or scald is extensive, immerse the whole limb or body in a bath of warm water to which ½ lb. of soda (or washing-soda) has been added for each gallon of water in the bath. But first, give the patient Urtica Urens (5 pilules every hour, or oftener if the pain is severe). Do not attempt to remove clothing if it is sticking to the burn; simply cut it away round the burn, removing as much as possible.

For burns caused by corrosive alkalis such as caustic soda, bathe with *vinegar* (1 tablespoonful in a cupful of water), or with raw tomato juice, or with cold tea. In an emergency, if you have nothing else handy, apply white of egg, or honey, to any kind of burn, and cover with lint and a bandage.

BITES AND STINGS OF INSECTS. If stung by a bee, remove the sting, squeezing it out or levering it out with a watch-key if you have one; then apply raw onion juice or vinegar. A wasp sting should be bathed with a solution of bicarbonate of soda (or washing soda) using a teaspoonful to a ¼ pint of water. If stung in the mouth, use the solution double strength, and hold it in the mouth for as long as possible. Apply hot cloths to the front of the throat.

The following remedies should also be kept in the house:

SLIPPERY ELM food-beverage, for gastric and intestinal inflammation, diarrhoea, etc., Slippery elm powder, for poultices. (From a health-foods shop.)

GUM-ARABIC for diarrhoea, dysentery, catarrhal conditions, gastritis, fevers, etc. (From a herbal supplier.)

ELDERFLOWER HERB, PEPPERMINT, AND COMPOSITION POWDER, for colds and feverish states, to encourage sweating. (From a herbal supplier.)

CINNAMON (pills) for flu, fevers, bowel cleansing, etc. (From a homoeopathic chemist.)

VEGETABLE CHARCOAL tablets, for flatulence, and indigestion. (From any chemist.)

SPIRITS OF CAMPHOR, for collapse, shock, or heart-attack. The dose is 3 drops in sweetened water. Applied to the neck and head, for headache. (Obtain from homoeopathic chemist.)

CAMPHORATED OIL, for massage of the chest and back in bronchial troubles.

THE THREE OILS (Camphorated oil 2 parts, olive oil 2 parts, and oil of turps. 1 part, mixed in a bottle) for application to all forms of rheumatic pain. (From any chemist.)

EXTRACT OF WITCH-HAZEL, OR FERRUM-PERCHLORIDE, for nose-bleeding. Apply on cotton-wool. (From any chemist.)

BELLA-DONNA tincture, or OIL OF CLOVES, for toothache. Apply to the tooth (neat).

CIDER-VINEGAR, for suspected food-poisoning. Place one tea-spoonful in a glassful of water, and take sips of the mixture every 5 minutes. (For other uses, see 'Cider-vinegar', page 244.)

FRIAR'S BALSAM (Tincture of benzoin), for inhalation to relieve congested nasal and bronchial passages; also for applying (neat) to unbroken chilblains.

CASTOR OIL, for dropping into the eye to soothe pain caused by a foreign body or other harmful substance such as acid. It is also taken internally as a remedy for food-poisoning (it should follow an emetic which has caused vomiting). Cider-vinegar (without an emetic) is an alternative remedy. Castor oil should *not* be taken if there is acute pain in the abdomen, or suspected appendicitis, but it can be taken (a tablespoon-ful in a lemon drink at bedtime) for prolonged stoppage of the bowels, and in brandy for prolonged diarrhoea. It can be applied to swellings and lumps of all kinds (including bunions), which it will reduce if used regularly for several weeks. It will also get rid of skin blemishes and wrinkles if gently smoothed in, with the finger-tips, every night at bed-time. For rheumatic joints, it should be mixed with olive oil and oil of turpentine, and applied externally, or Olbas oil can be used.

OLBAS OIL has many uses. It is indispensable in every home, for aches and pains of every kind, for coughs, colds, catarrh, etc. (From health-foods shop.)

LINSEED-OIL is an excellent bowel-lubricant; so, too, are the seeds (linseed) from which it is extracted. The seeds swell up when they reach the large bowel, and they have the power of attracting water, with the result that the contents of the large bowel are moistened and pushed on by the bulky mass of the seeds, and thus rendered easier of expulsion from the body. Linseed is also used for linseed tea, which is an excellent remedy for chest troubles (see 'Herbal Recipes'). It is also used for hot poultices. (Obtainable from any good chemist.)

LEMONS AND ONIONS should always be kept in the house. Lemon juice (neat) mixed with a pinch of common salt, can be taken in teaspoonful doses, every half hour or so, for biliousness. Lemon juice and 3 cloves in hot water, with a little added honey, is a good remedy for coughs and colds. Lemon juice applied to painful joints, bunions, and growths on the surface of the body (including cancerous growths) is very soothing. If a fish-bone gets stuck in the throat, raw lemon juice will slowly dissolve it. It will also cut through a diphtheria membrane if one forms in the throat. Onion juice is useful for applying to insect bites and wasp stings, and a cut onion is useful for placing on saucers around a sick room, to disinfect the air. To suck a bit of raw onion, or inhale the smell of a cut onion, will sometimes help to scotch an impending cold. Homoeopathic Allium cepa (onion) pilules will relieve a streaming head-cold.

FIREWEED ointment, for smearing on sore or inflamed eyes; also for cysts on the eyelid.

TINCTURE OF MYRRH for application to unbroken chilblains; also for massage in muscle-cramp, and for sore tongue or gums.

VINEGAR mixed with an equal quantity of water, can be used as a skin-freshener. In feverish conditions, the whole body should be sponged over with it. An extra-strong (acetic acid) vinegar (made by Coutts), obtainable from any good chemist, is used for massage of the spine, to tone up the whole nervous system.

Other emergency and first-aid remedies are given in *Homoeopathy for the First-Aider* by Dr. Dorothy Shepherd (Health Science Press).

COMMON AILMENTS
AND THEIR SPECIFIC TREATMENT

Mental or emotional stress, especially worry, upsets the glands in the stomach that produce the digestive acids, causing them to be over-active and to produce too much acid. A disturbed mind nearly always produces a disturbed digestive system, and the only real cure is to get rid of whatever is causing the disturbed mind.

Sometimes, however, dyspepsia is due to faulty feeding on deficiency foods, and to the eating of incompatible foods at the same meal. Also sometimes it is due simply to insufficient mastication of starch and sugar foods, which are partly digested by saliva in the mouth. Saliva is alkaline, and a piece of bread, well masticated, will cause a copious flow of saliva which will neutralize over-acidity of the stomach.

The intake of acid-forming foods (flesh foods, starch and sugar foods, and animal fats) should be reduced, and the intake of alkaline-forming foods (raw vegetable-juices, especially potato juice) increased. Casilan, a dried and powdered milk-protein, can replace animal-protein.

Sugar, and sugar-starch mixtures such as cakes, biscuits, etc., also jams, sweets, and chocolate, are acid-forming. Sugar should be replaced by pure honey; stick liquorice, dates, and raisins, can replace sweets.

Ordinary tea should be replaced by camomile-herb mixed with peppermint herb; ordinary coffee by dandelion coffee.

Table-salt and condiments should be replaced by garlic powder (garlic assists digestion); white bread and white flour by wholewheat bread and flour; flesh foods by milk-protein (Casilan).

Chewing a small piece of stick-liquorice after a meal encourages the outflow of saliva in the mouth, and this, being alkaline, helps to neutralize the over-acidity of the stomach. Vegetable-charcoal tablets, with, or after, meals are also helpful. They absorb stomach-gases, which give rise to acid eructations. Papain-compound tablets, made from the juice of the papaya fruit (known as the paw-paw in some parts of the world), which contains a powerful digestive enzyme, are even better (see *Appendix*). Lemon juice (1 dessertspoonful in hot water taken 2 hours after food) is sometimes helpful. Fried foods, cooked protein foods, and cooked foods containing fats should all be avoided.

In between meals, biochemic Nat. phos. pilules should be taken; allow 3 pilules to dissolve slowly under the tongue, 3 times a day. A pinch of Glaubers salts (Nat. sulph.) should be taken in a little hot water every morning, half an hour before food. Once a week, 2 pilules of homoeopathic sulphur 200 should be taken at bedtime, for 6 weeks. The herbal remedy is a tea made with 1 oz. Meadowsweet herb, ½ oz. dandelion root, ¼ oz. peppermint, and 1 pint boiling water. Infused for 20–30 minutes. Drink ¼ pint before meals.

ACNE

This skin trouble is common among teenagers. It is largely due to glandular changes that are taking place; these tend to upset the chemistry of the blood – although, if the blood were in a really clean and healthy condition, the trouble would be less likely to develop.

The first aim of treatment, therefore, is to purify the blood, and one of the best ways of doing this is by taking homoeopathic sulphur (in the 30th potency) for 3–4 weeks. The dose is 5 pilules night and morning. The following blood-purifying mixture should also be taken:

Fluid extract of echinacea	1 oz.
Fluid extract of yellow dock	1 oz.
Fluid extract of blue flag	1 oz.

The dose is 30 drops, in 1–2 tablespoonfuls of hot water, 3 times a day, before meals.

The diet should be one that includes plenty of fresh fruit, salads, and raw vegetable-juices (especially nettles, dandelion leaves, garlic, and watercress). A little unsalted butter may be eaten on wholewheat bread or toast, but margarine and cooking-fats (and all foods containing them) should be avoided. Fried foods, all sugar, sweets, chocolate, jams, cakes, pastry, pies, etc. should also be avoided. Wholewheat bread and wheatgerm should replace white bread, and honey or molasses should replace sugar, jams, and marmalade. A desire for sweet things can be satisfied by eating dates, raisins, grapes, and other sweet fruits rich in natural fruit-sugar. Camomile herb-tea helps to cleanse the blood.

Yoghourt or plantmilk should replace cream and custard on fruit. Kelp powder should replace table-salt, and all salted foods should be avoided. Salad-dressing should be made with a cold-pressed vegetable oil (such as sunflower seed oil) and cider-vinegar (equal quantities). Wheatgerm oil capsules (3 a day) should be taken; also 1 vitamin B12 tablet and 2 vitamin A capsules (with food).

The above diet, plus the homoeopathic remedies, should ensure a daily bowel movement, but, if it does not, take a teaspoonful of tincture of rhubarb at bedtime. Alternatively, a heaped teaspoonful of Epsom salts may be taken in $\frac{1}{2}$ pint of hot water on rising in the morning, but for the rest of that day no solid food should be ingested, only hot drinks. To start treatment with a thorough cleansing of the bowels is absolutely essential. Take prunes or prune juice for breakfast.

For suppurating blackheads, use Rumex ointment (see *Appendix*). If they are not suppurating, treatment with the rays of an ultra-violet-light lamp 2–3 times a week, is suggested, and thorough cleansing of the skin with Cetrimide, an antiseptic cleanser, at night, and in the morning.

Lemon juice applied 2–3 times a day is sometimes helpful.

ADENOIDS AND TONSILS (enlarged)

The purpose of tonsils, which are lymph-glands, is to filter harmful germs and their toxins out of the bloodstream. The tonsils are a first line of defence, and seldom, if ever, is it advisable or necessary to remove them surgically. If they become enlarged, they can usually be normalized by natural means, i.e. by correct feeding, combined with bowel-cleansing, skin stimulation, and breathing exercises.

Treatment. This should start with a 2-day fast on juices only. At bedtime, 1 teaspoonful dose of syrup of figs or of rhubarb tincture, should be given. The fast should be followed by 5 days on fruit and yoghourt – nothing else, except drinks of boiled water if thirsty. A dose of rhubarb may be needed every 3–4 days, to keep the bowels regular.

Gradually, after a week, the diet can be augmented, so that it includes salads and green vegetables every day, baked potatoes, wholewheat bread, a little farmhouse or cottage or lactic-acid cheese, nut-foods, soya-beans, lentils, and new-laid eggs. Sugar, sweets, chocolate, cakes, pastries, and starchy foods (especially packet cereals, mushed up with sugar and milk) should be omitted. Sugar and sweets should be replaced by honey, and dates; packet cereals by 'muesli' made of wheatgerm, barley-kernels, raisins, dates, and ground-up nuts; lots of fresh fruit, and drinks of fresh orange juice should replace tea, coffee, and milk.

Parents are often too anxious to fatten their children and encourage them to drink a lot of milk. This is unwise, because over-stimulation of body-growth during the growing years tends to shorten the life-span. Also, too much cow's milk increases the tendency (if there is one) to catarrh. Plant-milk is superior to pasteurized cow's milk. Flesh foods are not necessary and are better omitted. (See 'How to be healthy on a vegetarian diet', page 229.)

The throat should be gargled night and morning with lemon juice in warm water, some of which can be swallowed. Occasionally, it should be sprayed with tincture of Hydrastis (5 drops in $\frac{1}{4}$ pint of warm water). Fresh air to breathe at all times is more important, and stuffy rooms must be avoided. Powdered bayberry-bark should be used as snuff.

Daily exercise in the fresh air and plenty of sleep are both essential. A pad of some soft material should be squeezed out of cold water, bandaged on lightly over the tonsil area before going to bed at night, and kept on all night.

Dr. Compton-Burnett's booklet *Enlarged tonsils cured by medicine* (Health Science Press) should be read. His homoeopathic remedies can be taken alternately with Dr. Gilbert's biochemic remedy T.111 (see *Appendix*).

ANAEMIA

A blood-test will show that this is an impoverished state of the blood, the number of red blood-cells which carry oxygen from the lungs to all parts of the body being much smaller than it should be. The result is a shortage of oxygen all over the body, with consequent tiredness, headaches, physical weariness, possibly slight fever, increase in the heart beat, and general malaise. A lack of red blood-cells can be caused by loss of them due to severe bleeding, destruction of them by poisons (lead, malarial poisons, etc.) and by self-produced antibodies; this process is called 'auto-immunity' (see 'Ulcerative Colitis' where it is fully explained). The manufacture of new red blood-cells can also be stopped by exhaustion of the bone-marrow which makes them. But the commonest cause of anaemia is 'deficiency' feeding, i.e. a diet deficient in first-class protein, in green vegetables, and in the B vitamins, especially B.12. Such a diet leads to general debility of the whole body, this leads to impoverishment of the blood, which leads to further debility. Thus a vicious circle is set up.

Treatment should therefore aim at a regeneration of the whole system, by means of correct feeding, a replacement of iron, copper, calcium, the B vitamins, and all other deficiencies, combined with rest, fresh air, and exercise.

However, anaemia is *not always* due to a poor diet: it *can* be caused by poor absorption of a nutritionally-good diet, brought about by a lack of digestive acids in the stomach – of hydrochloric acid and ascorbic acid (vitamin C), both of which are essential for the absorption of iron, copper, and calcium, all of which are essential for the manufacture of new red blood-cells in the bone-marrow. In other words, if stomach acids are lacking, iron and copper will not be absorbed from one's food, and new cells cannot be made by the bone-marrow.

To remedy the acids-deficiency, a capsule of glutamic-acid hydrochloride should be taken before meals, and 3 vitamin C capsules *with* meals. Brewers yeast (powder) should also be taken with meals. This is rich in all the B vitamins, especially folic acid, and will help digestion and absorption. Green leafy vegetables are also rich in folic acid, and should be eaten every day.

Iron is necessary for the formation of haemoglobin, the pigment in red blood-cells that carries oxygen from the lungs to all parts of the body. People whose blood lacks iron have a haemoglobin deficiency; this means that they suffer from oxygen starvation, which leads to a deterioration of all their tissues and organs, to debility and fatigue.

The oxidation of animal fats produces hydrogen-peroxide, and this destroys red blood-cells; so people with anaemia should cut down their intake of such fats, and step up their intake of vitamin E. This all-important vitamin breaks down the hydrogen-peroxide, as soon as it is formed, into oxygen and water, thus preventing its destruction of red cells.

Vitamin B.12 is closely bound to protein, and, before the body can make use of it, it must be set free from protein, by digestion. But the digestive powers of anaemic people are usually weak, so they are unable to set free the vitamin – hence their vitamin B.12 deficiency. To remedy this, they should take either vitamin B.12 tablets (1 a day is sufficient) or 2 teaspoonfuls of a preparation called 'Bio-Nektarin' after meals. This contains vitamin B.12, also iron in an easily-assimilable form. Foods containing traces of vitamin B.12 include soya-bean and all its derivatives, egg-yolk, plantmilk (which is made from soya-bean) alfalfa herb-tea, alfalfa tablets, Iceland moss. Dried liver (in tablet or powder form) contains all the B vitamins, including vitamin B.12. For non-vegetarians, this is the best remedy.

Animal fats should be largely replaced by vegetable fats. Margarine made of safflower-seed oil or sunflower-seed oil is an excellent substitute for butter. The diet should contain the following foods:

Wholewheat bread, wheatgerm, bran (Allinsons make a finely ground one), wheatgerm oil on salads and vegetables, nuts and seeds including almonds, hazel nuts, Brazil nuts, millet, sesame seed, sunflower seeds, lentils, soya-bean milk (dried and powdered, it is called Granogen), honey, molasses (rich in potassium), black treacle, sultanas, raisins, Spanish figs (when obtainable), sun-dried apricots, dates, apples, black grapes, green leafy vegetables and salads. These should include nettles (when young and succulent), turnip-tops, beetroots, onions, carrots, parsley, etc. Half a teacupful of raw *vegetable* juices (mixed), together with 3 kelp tablets, 3 alfalfa tablets, a little garlic powder or 2 garlic perles, plus a small teaspoonful of a yeast extract (such as salt-free Barmene) should be taken 2–3 times a day, between meals.

The herbal remedy is a tea made by simmering together in 2 pints of water, for 20–30 minutes, equal quantities of common garden sage, wild thyme, camomile, and gentian-root. A wineglassful of this should be taken with a trickle of honey, 2–3 times a day, between meals.

An excellent proprietary remedy, made by Parke Davis and Co., is Potassium and Lecithin tablets. Another is Eastons Syrup (rich in iron) and yet another, already mentioned, is Bio-Nektarin.

Pernicious Anaemia. This is due to the stomach's inability to produce 'intrinsic factor', a protein formed in the stomach, without which vitamin B.12 cannot be assimilated. Sometimes this inability is the result of a surgical operation on the stomach, but usually the lack of intrinsic factor is due to the fact that the stomach simply stops producing it, for no apparent reason. It has been suggested that 'auto-immunity' may be the reason. (For an explanation of auto-immunity, see 'Ulcerative Colitis'.) The remedy is vitamin B.12 with 'intrinsic factor' (injections are usually given).

Other causes of anaemia are: Tuberculosis (sometimes), Cancer (sometimes), Kidney disease.

ANGINA PECTORIS

This is often called neuralgia of the heart, for that is what it really is. It can be greatly relieved by improving the circulation of the nerves in the spinal cord which supply the chest and heart. To do this, apply a hot cloth or towel wrung out in very hot water, to the upper half of the spinal column, allowing it to remain there for 2–3 minutes. Repeat the application 5–6 times, and follow it with one cold application, and then some really deep massage of the muscles on both sides of the spine.

Sometimes pain in the chest region is caused by one of the spinal vertebrae being out of alignment. This can be easily diagnosed and rectified by a competent osteopath or chiropractor.

The general circulation can be improved, and the work of the heart relieved, by taking vitamin E capsules (see 'Circulatory Disturbances'). Take also vitamin B.12 tablets (1 a day), Calcium-plus tablets (3 a day), and rose-hip or acerola (3 with meals).

Homoeopathic Cactus grandiflorus 3x. should be taken every day, either in the form of fresh-plant tincture, or pilules (whichever is most convenient). The dose is 5 drops of the tincture in a teaspoonful of water before meals, or 5 pilules, dissolved slowly in the mouth, at bedtime.

Mag. Phos. 30x. should also be taken (5 pilules once a day), and ¼ teaspoonful of Epsom salts (Mag. Sulphate) in early-morning tea is advisable, as sometimes there is a lack of magnesium salts in the blood. The herbal remedy is Sarsaparilla root.

For the relief of a painful attack, apply hot cloths over the region of the heart, give smelling-salts composed of trichlorethylene, and a dose of spirits of camphor (2 drops in a little hot water sweetened with honey. It should be sipped slowly). When sweating starts, change to biochemic Mag. Phos. 6x. (5 pilules dissolved in a little hot water) and sip this till the pain eases. (Repeat as often as necessary.) Immersing the forearms in hot water is helpful.

APPENDICITIS

If digestion is normal, and if there is no over-eating of the wrong foods and no constipation, inflammation of the appendix cannot develop. If it does develop, and if an abscess forms, it can be cured without an operation – by fasting. An operation is a quicker cure, but peritonitis may follow it, and adhesions often form, and they are troublesome for the rest of your life; they can be relieved only by a second (and sometimes even a third) operation. However, a homoeopathic doctor should be called, for advice and treatment. (He will probably prescribe Baptisia (20 drops hourly) or Iris. 3x. every 2 hours.)

Nature-cure treatment of appendicitis permits no food for so long as the sufferer's temperature remains above normal. He (or she) is fed for the first few days on water only (it is taken in sips, one spoonful at a time), and is kept very quiet and warm, in a well-ventilated room. No aperient should be given, but, if an enema can be borne without too much discomfort, the lower bowel should be washed out with plain warm water (previously boiled), or an injection made into the rectum of 1 tablespoonful of pure olive oil. Hot compresses (i.e. cloths wrung out in hot elderflower tea), or hot bran poultices, should be applied to the seat of pain, as often as possible, and hot elderflower tea can be sipped instead of water. A recipe for the tea can be found under 'Herbal Recipes'.)

About the third day, the pain and discomfort should have eased sufficiently for a 2–3 pint enema of plain warm water to be given daily. Fresh fruit juices can then be taken, as well as elderflower tea, and, as soon as the temperature is down to normal and the pain has gone, an all-fruit diet can be taken, followed gradually by a return to normal diet.

Acupuncture, a method of treating disease first used by the Chinese over 5,000 years ago, has recently been revived and has been used with some success in the treatment of acute, *and* chronic, appendicitis. (See Dr. Korth's book *Some Unusual Healing Methods*, Health Science Press.)

ARTERIOSCLEROSIS (Hardening of the Arteries)

This usually precedes coronary thrombosis and heart troubles of all kinds, and the main cause is long years of incorrect feeding and deficiency foods. There should be a reduction in the intake of animal fats (butter, creamy milk, meat-fat, etc.), and an increase in the intake of vegetable fats, which are rich in E.F.A. (Essential Fatty Acids) and in Lecithin. These break up (emulsify) the globules of cholesterol in animal-fats, and keep them on the move, thus preventing blood-clots and the clogging of the blood-vessels, which obstructs the free flow of the blood to all the organs and tissues of the body.

Linoleic acid is the most important of the E.F.A., and the best source of it is safflower-seed oil, a little of which should be eaten every day. Sunflower seeds are perhaps the best source of vegetable fat because they are also rich in protein, minerals, and B vitamins, vitamins B and E being essential for proper use to be made of the fatty-acids. Other good sources of B vitamins are brewer's yeast and wheatgerm, both of which should be included in the daily diet, which, if it excludes flesh-foods, should include one tablet of vitamin B.12. Dried milk powder (Casilan) is a good substitute for flesh-foods, being rich in all the essential amino-acids, vitamins, and minerals. Sesame seeds and sunflower seeds also provide good vegetable-protein, in addition to calcium, iron and vitamins, including the all-important vitamin E.

Raw vegetable-juices are also an essential part of the daily diet. Beetroots and beetroot tops are especially beneficial, but cut away and discard the neck of the beetroot where the leaves sprout from. Three kelp tablets, 3 garlic perles, and 3 alfalfa tablets in a tablespoonful of hot water, should be added to $\frac{1}{4}$ cupful of the juices and sipped slowly before a meal.

Dandelion coffee should replace ordinary coffee, and rutin tea mixed with salus tea should replace ordinary tea, or be mixed with it (see *Appendix*).

Other (minor) causes of arteriosclerosis are:

1. An inherited tendency to it.
2. Emotional tension, and negative emotions such as fear and anger, which produces an excess of adrenalin and of cholesterol in the blood.
3. Poisons circulating in the bloodstream. These include lead (absorbed from water which is conducted through lead water-pipes, or from inhaling car-exhaust fumes) and nicotine from cigarette smoking.
4. Repeated infections with their bacilli and toxic products which damage the arterial walls.
5. Prolonged over-dosage with vitamin D or excessive sun-bathing in the nude, which produces an excess of vitamin D in the blood, with consequent sclerotic changes in the arterial walls.

ARTHRITIS

Inflammation of a joint or joints can have many causes, the chief of which are emotional tension or upset, faulty body-chemistry, and faulty feeding. It is thought that it can also be caused by auto-immunity. (For an explanation of auto-immunity, see 'Ulcerative Colitis'.)

Persistent nervous tension, anxiety, and emotional upsets cause changes in the pituitary-adrenal-gland relationship upsetting the balance of the various chemical secretions (hormones) produced by these glands. What happens is this: In the normal way, one of the hormones produced by the pituitary gland (its name is A.C.T.H.) stimulates the production by the adrenal glands of two hormones, one of which is called cortisone, the other is an inflammatory hormone. But if the secretion of A.C.T.H. is stopped or decreased by a neural blockage caused by a deep-seated emotional conflict or upset, the adrenal glands will cease production of enough cortisone to keep in check the inflammatory hormones it also produces. These inflammatory hormones will then set up inflammation in any strained or weakened parts of the body, particularly the muscles and joints and their internal capsular ligaments and membranes. For this reason, cortisone and A.C.T.H. are both used in the treatment of arthritis (they are injected into the blood-stream) to check the over-production of inflammatory hormones by the adrenal glands. These injections often do alleviate the symptoms, even though they do not cure. To cure, the cause must be removed. This is not too difficult if the cause is faulty body-chemistry or faulty feeding (deficiency foods, etc.), but not so easy if the main cause is an anxiety state or emotional tension. This can be cured only when the anxiety or tension is relieved.

Faulty body-chemistry can cause an insufficiency of acids hydrochloric and ascorbic) in the digestive juices of the stomach, and this means that, although you may be getting enough calcium in the foods you eat, you are not able to assimilate it properly because of a lack of these digestive acids, and it piles up in the joints. Thus, calcium is erroneously thought to be a cause of arthritic joints, whereas actually it is a *lack* of it in the blood that causes the trouble. A lack of calcium also means that vitamin C is deprived of help in forming good strong cartilage around the joints.

To remedy the deficiency of digestive acids (which tends to increase with age), a teaspoonful of cider-vinegar in a little warm water should be sipped before meals. This will make up any deficiency of hydrochloric acid, and, if an acerola tablet is taken with each meal, this will make up any deficiency of ascorbic acid. It will also supply vitamin C, without which calcium cannot be fully utilized by the body. One vitamin B.12 tablet, 3 vitamin A capsules, and 3 vitamin E capsules, should also be taken every day.

As for the meals themselves, the following foods should be avoided: all flesh foods, wheat bread and flour, white sugar products (jams, sweets, chocolates, etc.), strong tea and coffee, alcoholic drinks, table-salt and condiments. They should be replaced by: farmhouse cheese, cottage cheese, eggs, soya-bean milk, Casilan (powdered milk-protein), goats-milk yoghourt, food-yeast (powdered brewers yeast), nuts and seeds of all kinds including sunflower seeds, sesame seeds, linseed, millet, buckwheat seeds, pine-kernels; barley kernels, lentils and lentil flour, soya-beans and soya-bean flour; honey, molasses, black treacle, dates, maté tea, burdock-root tea, nettle tea, dandelion coffee, apple-juice (preferably home-made), kelp powder, garlic powder, celery powder. Wheatgerm can be included, but not wheat flour; rye bread or bread made with gluten-free flour (wheat starch) should replace it.

It is better that arthritics should keep to a gluten-free diet. It would, therefore, be advisable to cut out bread and other foods made of wheat-flour, because wheat contains much gluten. Gluten-free flour and gluten-free baking-powder can be obtained from Energen Foods Ltd. (Pound Lane, Willesden, London, N.W. 10).

A half cupful of raw vegetable-juices should be taken every day (before a meal), using potatoes, carrots, celery, cabbage, kale, and when available watercress, parsley, nettles, and dandelion leaves. Breakfast should consist of fresh ripe fruit (excluding citrus fruits, plums, and rhubarb) or sun-dried apricots, pears, or peaches, with a cupful of goat's milk yoghourt. It can be followed by a cup of dandelion coffee sweetened with molasses. A drink of the water in which beans *and* their pods have been cooked is a remedy that should be taken several times a day, between meals. When beans are out of season, they can be replaced by homoeopathic Phaseolus pilules (made from beans). Some of the best vegetable-juices are imported from Switzerland and are obtainable from most health-food shops.

The treatment should start with a short fast of 2–4 days, during which time only vegetable-juices, apple-juice, maté tea, tea made with nettles or burdock-root, and plain boiled water or Malvern spring-water, should be taken.

For the first 2 days, the bowels should be cleansed by taking at bedtime a teaspoonful dose of tincture of rhubarb in hot water, followed next morning by a teaspoonful of Epsom salts in ½ pint of hot water. This should be followed by a hot drink, and it should purge the bowels very thoroughly. The bowel movement is followed by a bath, using a bath-brush to friction the skin, but no soap, then a rub-down with rough towels, to produce a skin-glow. Then the painful joints should be massaged with warmed castor oil (or iodine oil) and manipulated gently but firmly, to keep them from getting immovable. Two or three times a week, a moderately hot bath, containing about a pound of common Epsom salts, should be sat in for 10 minutes. This helps elimination of toxins through the skin. No soap should be used.

Outdoor exercise is most important. Walking exercise will help the body to produce its own cortisone, and will oxygenate all the tissues and aerate the lungs. But, if exercise is not possible because too painful, massage of the limbs, the back, and the abdomen should be given daily, as well as manipulation of all the joints; also breathing and other simple exercises should be practised, many of which can be done in bed if the patient is not able to get up. These, and the inclusion in the diet of molasses, soaked figs and prunes, honey, yoghourt, All-bran, oatmeal, and wheatgerm cereal, Alpine-herb tea and maté tea, and a bi-weekly dose of tincture of rhubarb at bedtime, will help to keep the bowels regular. (Tincture of rhubarb is only a gentle laxative, but gives tone to the musculature of the bowel and is anti-rheumatic.) A glassful of Vichy water (hot) should be taken every morning, on waking, to help bowel action.

Rest, relaxation, and freedom from worry, anxiety, and tension, are an important part of the treatment. For this reason, if the patient can afford it, it is best for him (or her) to go and stay for a few weeks at a nature-cure establishment. This ensures that he gets proper diet without all the trouble of getting it (or of getting someone else to get it). It ensures proper rest and relaxation, and skilful manipulation of joints, together with massage, medicated baths, and, if necessary, bowel wash-outs given by skilled nurses. It is money well spent.

For 3 days before taking other remedies, 2 pilules of homoeopathic sulphur 6x. should be taken 3 times a day, between meals. Sulphur increases the efficacy of all subsequent remedies by its cleansing action on liver and intestines.

Biochemic remedies. Nat. phos. (sodium phosphate) 3 pilules before meals; Kali. phos. (potassium phosphate) 3 pilules after meals; Silica, 3 pilules at bedtime; a pinch of Glaubers salts (Nat. sulph.) in hot water or early-morning tea. (All pilules should dissolve slowly under the tongue.) Or take Dr. Gilbert's specific remedy for arthritis (D.128).

A good homoeopathic remedy for gouty arthritis with sore and aching feet is Ledum (Wild rosemary) taken in homoeopathic pilules. The feet of socks and stockings (a clean pair every day) should be sprinkled with flowers of sulphur. A hot foot-bath containing sea-salt will ease painful feet.

ASTHMA

Strictly speaking, asthma is not really a disease; it is simply a symptom of a disorder, but the fundamental cause of the disorder is as yet unknown. Until it *is* known, a cure is not possible; all that can be done is to treat the so-called causes of which asthma is the symptom. The commonest of these causes is a toxic state of the blood, usually due to faulty feeding and to kidney disfunction, the latter being aggravated by adrenal-gland inactivity. Other contributory causes are:

(*a*) Faulty breathing. This can be cured by learning to breathe low-down with your diaphragm instead of high-up with your chest muscles. Learning to do this will not be easy at first, as most asthmatics are chest-breathers, but it *must* be mastered, as the way you breathe is all-important. To practise breathing, sit propped up in a comfortable high-backed chair or bed; place your hands on your abdomen just above the navel and breathe in through your nose so that your hands rise with the upward movement of your abdomen and fall with it when it drops as you let go the breath. Only abdominal muscles should move – not the chest muscles.

(*b*) Indigestion and flatulence. Indigestion causes disturbance of the breathing apparatus, by pressing on the Vagus nerve, the nerve that controls not only the stomach but also the bronchial tubes. The pressure restricts the free flow of air into and out of the lungs, with consequent breathing difficulty. If therefore any of the suggested foods cause indigestion, omit them.

(*c*) Exposure to a particular substance can trigger off an attack. For example, eating a particular food to which you are allergic, or inhaling a particular dust or pollen in the atmosphere. An attack can also be caused by exposure to cold and damp air, or smoky air.

(*d*) Emotional upset or strain can trigger off an attack; it is not understood how or why.

(*e*) Some people have an inherited tendency to asthma.

Daily outdoor exercise is important, remembering to breathe low-down and to take care not to over-fill the lungs. Complete exhalation is more important than deep inhalation. Singing exercises are helpful; so, too, is manipulation of the upper part of the spine by a chiropractor.

To be really effective, diet-reform should be preceded by a short 2–3 day fast (or semi-fast) on fruit-juices and water, and an early-morning purging dose of Epsom salts should be taken to thoroughly cleanse the bowels of all toxic waste-materials. Diet-reform alone, without this preliminary cleansing treatment, is only a half-measure.

Salt, animal-fats, and over-refined carbohydrate foods such as white flour and white sugar, should be avoided. Meat can be replaced by farmhouse cheese, free-range eggs, nuts and seeds, soya-bean milk and yoghourt. Honey should replace sugar entirely, and sunflower-seed oil should replace animal fats for cooking. Instead of white bread and flour, eat wholewheat bread and flour; instead of sugar and jams, eat honey, molasses, black treacle, or malt-extract; instead of alcoholic drinks, drink apple-juice made at home in your own juice-press; instead of tea and coffee, drink dandelion coffee and comfrey-herb tea; instead of table-salt and condiments, use garlic powder, and kelp powder; instead of cow's milk, use plantmilk and (if obtainable) goat's milk.

The diet should consist largely of fresh vegetables and raw vegetable-juices; salads dressed with sunflower-seed oil (or soya-bean oil) and cider-vinegar; avoid acid fruit; eat sun-dried fruit (apricots, peaches, pears, figs and dates). Carrots, onions, spinach and beetroot are especially valuable, because they are rich in *vitamin A*, a vitamin that is most important to asthmatics. Other foods rich in vitamin A are: fish-liver oil, liver, watercress, butter, corn oil, cheese, eggs, peas, carrots and apricots.

All aluminium cooking vessels, kettles, teapots, etc. should be discarded and replaced by stainless steel or enamel.

Shower baths are beneficial. This is because water, falling from a height, bombards the body with 'negative ions' as it descends. A hot Epsom salt bath once or twice a week should be followed by a cool shower-bath, if possible.

An attack can be relieved by administering adrenaline, and by a hot foot-bath; by applying hot cloths to the chest, and by inhaling the smoke from burning coffee-beans or dried nettles or from burning propolis (a sort of bees-wax).

For wheezing, put one teaspoonful of cider-vinegar into a teacupful of warm water and take frequent sips of it.

A remedy that never fails to give relief is onion-juice mixed with honey. To prepare it (overnight), lay thin slices of raw onion on a plate; spread honey on them; cover with a basin or soup plate, and allow to stand all night. The resulting juice should be taken in teaspoonful doses whenever the cough is troublesome. A similar syrup containing garlic can be bought from most chemists; lemon juice in hot water, with honey, is also helpful.

Other important remedies that should be taken daily (with meals) are: Vitamin A capsules (3 a day), vitamin E capsules (3 a day), vitamin B.12 (1 tablet), rose-hip or acerola tablets (2 with each meal), Calcium-plus tablets (3 a day), garlic capsules (1 with meals).

The herbal remedy is a tea made with Euphorbia herb (Asthma-weed) $\frac{1}{2}$ oz., Lungwort (1 oz.), Hyssop (1 oz.), Irish Moss ($\frac{1}{4}$ oz., pre-soaked), comfrey-herb (1 oz.), Horehound ($\frac{1}{2}$ oz.). Half these quantities to 1 pint of boiling water.

A homoeopathic remedy is Sambuccus niger 30x. (elderberry), 5 pilules at bedtime.

Biochemic. Nat. sulph. (3x.) and silica, 2 pilules of each, between meals.

Cardiac asthma is a symptom of heart failure. It should be treated with doses of homoeopathic Convallaria 3x. (2 pilules with meals).

At Driburg in Germany, the natural-spring waters are curative because they contain lime, iron, and sulphur, all of which are needed for the formation of blood-albumen, which has a great capacity for absorbing oxygen. *If the oxygen-content of the blood can be increased sufficiently, asthma can be greatly relieved, if not cured.*

The Driburg water can be synthesized by adding to one quart of distilled water the following: 15 grains sulphate of soda, 15 grains sulphate of lime, 15 grains sulphate of magnesia, 15 grains carbonate of lime, and $\frac{1}{2}$ grain carbonate of iron.

BACKWARDNESS IN CHILDREN

Foods and food-supplements that physically and mentally under-developed children should be given daily include the following:

Wheatgerm cereal to which is added 2 calcium-plus tablets and 2 rose-hip or acerola tablets (ground up in a nutmill), one teaspoonful of Yestamin powder (brewer's yeast), a tablespoonful of Granogen (soya-bean milk), a saltspoonful of wheatgerm oil, and a little plantmilk.

A wineglassful of raw vegetable-juices to which 3 kelp tablets, 3 alfalfa tablets (ground up), and a small teaspoonful of 'Vecon' have been added; bread, cakes, and biscuits made of wholewheat flour, not white flour; honey for all sweetening, instead of sugar, jam, etc.; dates instead of sweets; potatoes cooked in their skins; plenty of salads, fresh fruit, and sun-dried fruit (apricots, peaches, etc.).

Jellies, made at home with 'Gelozone' (Irish Moss) and fresh fruit juices, eaten with yoghourt or plantmilk. Plantmilk is purer than cow's milk, which nowadays contains many substances of doubtful value to humans. Like soya-bean milk, it contains vitamin B.12, the 'growth' vitamin.

BALDNESS

Massage the scalp frequently with equal parts of olive oil and oil of rosemary. Shampoo with extract-of-rosemary shampoo, using rainwater, if available. Sunlight (real or artificial) is sometimes very helpful. Artificial sunlight (ultra-violet light) treatment can be obtained at most hospitals. (See also 'Hair, Falling Out or Thinning'.)

Do not wear a hat; gradually harden the head to wind and rain and sunshine, starting in the summer.

BILIOUS ATTACK

Drink a small cup of black coffee containing lemon-juice and a pinch of common salt, and eat nothing for twenty-four hours; then eat only raw apples for a further twenty-four hours. The coffee must be made with genuine pure coffee without chicory; coffee-substitutes are useless.

A homoeopathic remedy is tincture of barberry (berberis), 5 drops in a tablespoonful of water, every 4 hours. (See 'Liver troubles'.)

BITES AND STINGS OF INSECTS

The pain and swelling caused thereby can be relieved by moistening and rubbing with raw onion, or one's own saliva.

BLADDER AND KIDNEY TROUBLES

Sufferers from bladder and kidney complaints should drink plenty of fluids, especially alpine-herb tea (which contains buchu, clivers, couch-grass, senna, etc.), parsley tea, and barley-water made with brown pot-barley. All drinking-water should be boiled, and, if the water-supply is fluoridated in your district, instal a Safari water-purifier, or drink only Malvern spring-water (obtainable from health-foods shops and some wine shops) – better still, live elsewhere (if you can), as fluoridated water is your worst enemy, and will prevent your complete recovery.

Intake of starch and sugar foods should be reduced, and flesh foods should be omitted altogether, as they contain prurines (the animals' waste-products), the elimination of which, in addition to your own, puts an extra burden on your kidneys.

Your diet should be salt-free, but, if salt *is* eaten, it should be Dr. Gilbert's Bio-salt. Kelp powder (dried seaweed) is a good substitute for salt. Honey should replace sugar entirely. Dandelion coffee should replace ordinary coffee. Vitamin A (3 capsules) should be taken daily with food.

No food, other than bananas, grapes, or raw apples, should be eaten before midday. A teaspoonful of cider-vinegar in a cup of hot water should be taken at bedtime, and the juice of half a lemon in $\frac{1}{2}$ pint of hot water on rising.

In a little book called *About the Grape Cure*, by Basil Shackleton, (Thorsons) the author tells how he cured himself of serious kidney trouble by living entirely on grapes and grape-juice for several weeks. A diet of bananas only, for 7–10 days, is indicated when kidney disfunction is causing uraemia (a surplus of urea in the blood).

A homoeopathic remedy for weakness of the kidneys, difficult urination, stone or gravel, is mother-tincture of barberry (berberis). The dose is 5 drops in a tablespoonful of water 3 times a day before meals. It can be sweetened with a trickle of honey. Alternatively, homoeopathic barberry 3x. pilules may be taken. The dose is 3 pilules (on the tongue) 3 times daily, half an hour before meals. Or take Dr. Gilbert's biochemic specific remedy for bladder and kidney troubles (see *Appendix*). Tincture of Solidago is Dr. Vogel's remedy.

Cystitis. (Inflammation of the bladder.) This is usually due to bacterial infection; but germs cannot live and multiply in a clean bloodstream. Cystitis could never arise, therefore, unless the blood were in an unclean state. Such a state is usually caused by faulty feeding and/or deficiency foods, by chronic constipation, or by previous drug-treatment of fevers, influenza, etc.

The orthodox treatment for cystitis is purely local treatment, i.e. bladder wash-outs with suppressive drugs. Such treatment completely ignores the fact that cystitis is a systemic ailment, and that local treatment fails, therefore, to tackle the real cause of the trouble – i.e. the unclean state of the blood. The treatment for this, as for all other inflammatory diseases caused by an impure bloodstream, is fasting on juices for as long as the acute symptoms and the pain last. Frequent drinks of alpine-herb tea, of elderflower-and-mint tea, of barley-water, and of grape-juice may also be taken, but no solid food. The pain and inflammation can be eased by sitting in hot water which reaches just up to the navel.

This hip-bath should be followed by a cold compress on the bladder region, repeated 2–3 times daily. A dose of Dr. Gilbert's specific remedy for cystitis should be taken every 4 hours, and a dose of 'Antitis' can also be taken at night (see *Appendix*). Sugar and sugar-products, also meat and alcohol, must be avoided.

Stone, Gravel, and Calculus. Usually, the formation of stones is due to a deficiency of oxygen and of mineral salts in the blood, and to an over-indulgence in meat. Meat-eaters, especially meat eaters who drink beer, wine, or spirits, the alcohol of which withdraws oxygen from the blood, need an abundance of oxygen for the complete digestion of animal flesh. Through insufficient oxygen, the constituents of the meat are not sufficiently oxidized into water, carbonic-acid gas, nitrogen, and urea, and the result of their partial oxidation is uric acid, which, unless a great deal of water is drunk instead of alcoholic drinks, forms into calculus, gravel, or stones. Plenty of oxygen is also required by the spleen for the formation of formic acid, which dissolves stones made of phosphate and oxalate of lime. The spleen is unable to produce the acid if the blood lacks oxygen.

The remedy, therefore, is to breathe fresh air at all times, to avoid sugar, flesh foods, and alcoholic drinks, and drink plenty of water (boiled). Malvern or natural-spring water is better than tap water.

Stone in the bladder. Stew gently for about an hour, 1 oz. Eupatorium herb, 1 oz. burnet-saxifrage herb, and 1 oz. bladderwrack, in 2 pints of water. Strain, and take a wine-glassful every 2–3 hours.

Stone in the kidney. A homoeopathic remedy is mother tincture of barberry. The dose is 5 drops in a tablespoonful of water 3 times a day before meals. The herbal remedy is a tea made of bladderwrack herb, buchu herb, parsley-piert, and parsley, using 1 oz. of each herb to 2 pints of water. Make fresh every day. When fresh parsley is not available, dried parsley can be used, though this is not so efficacious. (See *Appendix* for the recipe.) The water in which runner-beans are cooked (without salt) is also a good remedy. Grapefruit should be eaten daily.

Magnesium deficiency is related to kidney troubles, so, before breakfast, take ¼ teaspoonful of Epsom salts (Mag. sulph.) in a little hot water or unsweetened tea, and 3 Dolomite tablets with meals. Biochemic Mag. phos. 6x. can be taken as and when required for the pain. Dissolve 6 pilules in a little hot water and sip it slowly.

Other liquid remedies that are often effective in dissolving the stone are the juice of a lemon, or one teaspoonful of cider-vinegar, in hot water, 20 minutes before meals.

Keep to an all-fruit and vegetable diet, with drinks of the herb tea, lemonade, and cider, for a few days. This applies especially to people who are overweight. It should include pears, grapes, grapefruit, apples, onions, asparagus, leeks, carrots and vitamin A capsules (3 a day) with meals.

Abdominal exercises also help to reduce abdominal girth and to stimulate kidney activity. Try doing the following exercise:

Lie flat on the floor, toes tucked under the front edge of the wardrobe or other heavy piece of furniture, and from this position raise your head, shoulders, and trunk to sitting position without bending your knees. Repeat several times.

BLOOD-PURIFIERS

All green vegetables and salad crops, especially watercress, dandelion leaves, garlic, and nettles, are good blood-cleansers. Of the many herbs, echinacea is one of the best. The dried herb can be used, making it into tea, using 1 oz. of the herb to 1 pint of boiling water, but homoeopathic mother-tincture of echinacea is preferable. Its value is enhanced if 1 part of Hydrastis tincture is added to 4 parts of echinacea. Half a small teaspoonful of the mixture should be taken in a little hot water, 3 times daily, before meals.

A good herbal remedy is made of a mixture of the following herbs: Blue flag (1 oz.), yellow dock (1 oz.), echinacea (1 oz.), American mandrake ($\frac{1}{2}$ oz.). Cover with $1\frac{1}{2}$ pints of boiling water and gently simmer for 15 minutes. Then strain, and take 1 tablespoonful 3 times daily. Homoeopathic remedies include sarsaparilla, berberis, Iris, burdock-root, rhubarb root, red clover, allium sativum (garlic). Granatum 30 (Pomegranate) is the remedy for bowel-toxaemia. Any remedy should be preceded for 2 days by Sulphur 200 (2 pilules night and morning) and followed by Sulphur 30, for 2 weeks.

The 'macrobiotic' diet can with benefit be adopted for a period of from 5–10 days. It consists of cooked brown rice, topped with MISO sauce, and drinks of MU tea. (These foods can be obtained from The Macrobiotic Centre, 8a All Saints Road, London, W.11.) Miso sauce is made by Lima Products, and is obtainable from Hofels Pure Foods, but most health-foods shops stock it, also the MU tea.

Boils and Carbuncles

These should be regarded as beneficial and curative, being Nature's way of ridding the body of noxious poisons. The Greek physician Hippocrates induced boils artificially in those of his patients who were, in his opinion, suffering from toxaemia (self-poisoning), if their bodies lacked the vitality to produce such outlets naturally. See *Healing by Water* by T. Hartley Hennessey (C. W. Daniel Co., 60 Muswell Road, London, N.10) – 'Hydrotherapy' is a short summary of it.

To draw a boil or carbuncle to a head so that it bursts and discharges its toxins, spread equal parts of pure honey and cod-liver oil on a clean piece of white lint or linen. Apply this to the boil, cover with cotton-wool, and a piece of oiled silk, and secure in position with pieces of adhesive tape. The honey and oil dressing should be renewed every 8 hours.

The curative power of honey is due to its power to draw to

the site of the boil or carbuncle the body-fluids which contain 'anti-bodies' (germ-fighters). These anti-bodies, together with honey's own bactericidal power, overcome the infection.

To avoid frequent boils, keep to a cleansing diet consisting largely of fresh raw fruits, vegetables, vegetable-juices, and salads omitting sweet and starchy foods, and replacing fresh foods with farmhouse cheese, cottage cheese, free-range eggs, nuts and seeds (millet, sesame, sunflower seeds, etc.), lentils, soya-beans, and brewer's yeast.

Biochemic Ferrum phos. tablets, taken in the early stages, will sometimes ward off suppuration (the coming-to-a-head process); biochemic Silica will encourage it.

Fluid extract of echinacea	1 oz.
Fluid extract of American Mandrake	½ oz.

The dose is half a large teaspoonful in hot water, 3 times daily, before meals.

Homoeopathic Sulphur 30 should be taken at bedtime. The dose is 5 pilules.

BOWEL TROUBLES

See Diarrhoea, Constipation, Colitis.

BRAIN-FAG

Drink cowslip-herb tea to which a pinch of isinglass has been added (Brazilian isinglass is best). Take also biochemic Kali phos. (5 pilules at bedtime) and biochemic Calc. Phos. (5 pilules mid-morning).

BRIGHT'S DISEASE

The herbal remedy is milkweed-herb tea. The biochemic remedy is Calc. phos. (3 pilules, 3 times a day). There are many homoeopathic remedies; to find the right one for *you*, consult a homoeopathic doctor.

BRONCHIAL CATARRH

Slice an onion on a plate. Add to it one teaspoonful of pure honey. Cover with an inverted basin and leave for several hours. Take the resulting juice in teaspoonful doses. Garlic is as good as onion, if not better. A ready-to-use garlic preparation called 'Liquafruta' can be obtained from most chemists. It also contains liquorice and linseed, and other natural ingredients good for chest complaints.

BRONCHITIS AND BRONCHO-PNEUMONIA

The best way to cure both of these ailments is to fast, on juices only, for a day or two. A cup of hot elderflower-and-mint tea should be taken every half hour until sweating begins, then only every hour. The sweat should be removed with a dry towel. The elderflower tea can be alternated with comfrey tea, and with hot lemon drinks. The chest, throat, and back should be well massaged with Olbas oil, or with camphorated oil (warmed). Movements to mobilize the chest should be given, followed by a cold compress on the chest after the bedtime massage.

People with chronic bronchitis should follow the diet advice given for catarrh. A very helpful remedy is a tea made with equal quantities of the following: yarrow, coltsfoot, horehound, lungwort, aniseed, liquorice-stick, composition powder (or essence), peppermint essence ($\frac{1}{4}$ oz.) or peppermint herb ($\frac{1}{2}$ oz.). A ready-made fluid-extract of elderflowers, peppermint, and composition powder can be obtained from most health-foods shops.

BUNIONS

Paint with castor oil and iodine (mixed). Take homoeopathic Sulphur 6x. and sprinkle flowers of sulphur in the feet of socks or stockings.

CANCER

There are many varying opinions as to the cause(s) of cancer, but most scientists agree that it is a neoplastic disease, i.e. a disease characterized by abnormal and excessive cell-growth – in other words, cell-growth gone haywire. They all agree that treatment should aim at inhibition of abnormal cell-growth, and that treatment with plants in their natural state holds out more hope of success than treatment with synthetic man-made chemicals. This is because all chemical agents which destroy tumour-tissue destroy also healthy non-tumour tissue, whereas plant-extracts do not do so. (Some natural anti-tumour substances are given on page 80.)

The late Sir Arbuthnot Lane believed that cancer is the end-result of toxaemia – a retention of toxins in the blood. Such retention can be due to mental, emotional, or physical stress and strain; to wrong feeding and a poor diet; to poisonous chemicals in and on our foods and water; and to incomplete elimination of waste-products and toxins because of the inefficiency of our eliminative organs.

Professor Enderlein, the cancer expert of Berlin University, believes that the eating of flesh foods is one of the main causes of cancer, and the late Mr. Kasper Blond, F.R.C.S., an eminent cancer specialist, and author of 'Liver damage as a cause of cancer', considered that cancer is a degeneration of body-tissues caused by damage to the liver through long years of faulty feeding and of incomplete elimination of waste-products. He, too, condemned the eating of flesh foods, because, he said, they are never *completely* digested, and the undigested portions go rotten in the bowel and produce poisons damaging to the liver. He maintained that a diet free from animal-protein is the most important factor in the regeneration of a damaged liver – that a damaged liver *is* capable of regeneration if further damage by incorrect eating can be avoided, and that the lives of cancer sufferers can be prolonged indefinitely if they eat whole natural foods supplemented by biochemic 'tissue' salts – potassium nitrates, in particular.

Mr. Blond considered that cancer is a nutritional and a social problem, not a medical one – in other words, that it is a problem of 'prevention'. 'Prevention', he says, 'would be possible if the millions spent on drugs, operations, irradiations, etc. in hospitals were used for improving food-production and food-distribution, and for the spread of knowledge concerning nutrition.' He believed that disease of all sorts (including cancer) could be prevented if whole natural foods, grown in naturally-fertilized soil free of added chemicals and poisonous sprays, were the only kind available.

If they were, the food industrialists, who make big money out of turning whole natural foods into fragmented unnatural ones, would be deprived of their livelihood; thus it is that the health of the nation is really in the hands of 'vested interests' whose only concern is to make money, not to prevent ill-health and disease. There is nothing that the medical profession can do about it. It is up to the Government to do more than it *is* doing.

On the subject of meat-eating, Mr. Blond says, 'Man is the only animal who cooks food before eating it. It is likely that cooking renders meat unsuitable for assimilation, because cooking destroys its vitamins and enzymes, and these are necessary for its digestion and assimilation.' He continues, 'The prevention of liver-damage is the main problem (in cancer). The second problem is the regeneration of an already damaged liver. I am convinced that a diet free from animal protein is the most important factor in such regeneration. No incurable disease exists, for Nature can cure them all, including cancer.' Mr. Blond advises all doctors who are treating cancer patients to read Dr. Hay's books *A New Health Era*, and *Health via Food* (see book-list at the end of this book). Dr. Hay's advice to cancer sufferers is to eat all foods in their raw state, as far as possible. They should also include wheatgerm, dried liver tablets, brewer's yeast, acerola or rose-hip tablets, yoghourt, vitamin E, and 1–2 teaspoonfuls of cold-pressed oil (wheatgerm or safflower).

The late Sir Robert McCarrison, eminent nutritionist and joint-author with Dr. Hugh Sinclair of *Nutrition and Health*, stated that, in the absence of vitamins (or if they are under-supplied), neither proteins, carbohydrates, fats, nor salt, are properly utilized by the body – that they are largely wasted – and that, deprived of its vitamins and enzymes, meat-protein yields products harmful to the organism. This view supports the belief of many investigators that chronic diseases (including cancer) are diseases of civilized countries – presumably because, in civilized countries, food (including flesh-food) is cooked before it is eaten, and cooking destroys its vitamins and digestive enzymes.

Dr. Joseph Issells, a pioneer in the treatment of long-standing cancer cases, established a private clinic at Rottach-Egern am Tegernsee, near Munich (now closed), where the first step in his treatment was to eliminate focal infections (such as septic tonsils and teeth). He then corrected nutrition. He also emphasized the importance of keeping the blood slightly alkaline, of excluding flesh-foods from the diet and of eating raw foods.

Dr. Holman, bacteriologist, of Cardiff Infirmary, emphasizes the importance of a good oxygen intake. He says that a lack (or a diminished supply) of oxygen may be connected with the high incidence of cancer – that the more actively oxygenated our bodies, the better we shall be able to combat the toxic substances we ingest with our foods and from the air, which adversely influence our normal body-cells.

It is thought that cancer can be caused by a lack of oxygen in the blood, because, without enough oxygen, residual wastes of cell-activity are not burnt up (all fires need oxygen to make them burn brighter), and these wastes accumulate in the intercellular spaces and interfere with cell-respiration and cell-function.

Writing on cancer in *Mother Earth*, the Journal of The Soil Association, in January 1962, Dr. Holman says:

The greatest problem in medicine which faces us today is the disease called cancer. This is the result of chronic interference with the fundamental catalase-peroxide mechanism of our body cells, brought about by our own folly.

The answer to this disease is to have all our efforts focused on the *preventive* aspect. To this end it is urgently required that a concerted effort be made, at international level, to curtail the intake of catalase-inhibiting agents, whether in the air, foods, drinks, drugs, or radiation to which we are exposed.

This plan should be coupled with a campaign to increase the intake of catalase by the consumption of fresh, living foodstuffs, together with a re-education of man to use his animal body in the way for which it was designed. Cancer prevention can show results – if we pull together and reform some of the bad habits so prevalent in our civilized way of living.

(Catalase is a digestive ferment, produced by, and essential to, living organisms (plants, animals, and Man). It can initiate, accelerate, or retard a chemical change, without itself becoming changed in any way.)

So the plan of attack for the prevention of cancer should be threefold:

1. It should aim to increase our intake of catalase, by encouraging people to eat whole fresh foods (wholegrains, fresh fruit, and fresh vegetables, all of which are rich in catalase) instead of tinned, bottled, packeted, and other dead foods, which are devoid of catalase. (Meat, of course, is not only a dead food but it also contains extractives, i.e. poisonous nitrogenous waste-materials, such as urine, which were on their way out of the animal when it was killed.)

2. It should aim to increase the manufacture of catalase by our own body cells, by telling people not only to eat

natural whole foods which encourage the growth of catalase in the cells, but to take outdoor muscular exercise every day, a lack of which leads to a decrease of the catalase content, as also of the oxygen content, of the cells.

3. It should aim to curtail the ingestion of agents which destroy or inhibit catalase. These agents are fume-laden and smoke-laden air, which pollutes the oxygen so vital to the 'burning-up' or purifying processes of the body. Other agents which destroy or inhibit the production of catalase are chlorine and fluorine which are added to drinking water; drugs, serums, and vaccines of all kinds (including anti-biotics, aspirin, etc.); chemicals used in all types of preserved foods (shop bread and cakes, bottled and tinned fruit and fruit juices, tinned vegetables, etc.); artificial fertilisers and poisonous insecticides and sprays used on crops and vegetables, also on grass eaten by cows and sheep. (If we eat the flesh of these animals, these poisonous substances get into our bodies.)

In his books *Simpler and Safer Remedies* and *Victory over Cancer* (Athene Publishing Co.), Cyril Scott (nutritionist) says that, after long years of studying the problem, he has come to the conclusion that one of the primary causes of cancer and other morbid growths is a deficiency of potassium in the blood.

Possible secondary causes may be (1) irritants, such as oil-tars in smoke-laden air, (2) chemicals in and on our foods and our water supply, (3) tobacco-tars from the smoking habit, (4) the use of aluminium cooking vessels, and of baking-powder (which contains alum).

He bases his conclusions on the fact that plants, trees, and animals, as well as human beings, develop morbid growths. In the case of a plant or a tree, the growth takes the form of an unsightly excrescence, but, because a plant or a tree has no vital organs, this does not kill it. In the case of a human being it sometimes *does*; anyway it is a threat to life.

He goes on to say 'the orthodox treatment is to burn the growth away with rays, or to cut it out with the knife, but, as neither of these drastic measures gets rid of the real cause of the trouble, but merely deals with the effect, another growth may, sooner or later, form, because scarred tissue provides a fertile soil for such tumours. In other words, burning or cutting cannot make good a potash deficiency in the blood, hence the recurrence.'

A shortage of potassium in the body can arise for several reasons:

1. Our foods may be lacking in potassium if grown in potassium-deficient soil, or if (in the case of vegetables) all the potassium is boiled out of them and thrown away in the cooking-water.
2. We lose potassium every day, in our excretions, in our cast-off cells, in our urine, etc. and by our habit of eating common salt which destroys potassium.
3. Long-continued local irritations, also worry, rob the blood of potassium, and, unless this is made good by eating natural unrefined foods which are rich in potassium, growths or arthritis (or both) are likely to occur.

Mr. Scott goes on to say that neurotic people often worry about cancer – that he, as a young man, suffered from a fear of morbid growths, and that only when he came to study the whole question of diet did he lose that fear. He believes that a correct diet consisting of whole natural foods rich in minerals, especially potassium, is the answer to the cancer problem. He advises everyone to avoid white flour products, white sugar, boiled vegetables (unless the vegetable water is also ingested), salty foods, etc. He advises a teaspoonful of crude black molasses, which is very rich in potassium, every day.

The late Dr. Forbes-Ross, author of *Cancer, its Genesis and Treatment*, recommended a pinch of bicarbonate of potash to be taken every morning in hot water, before breakfast, as a precaution against growths of all kinds.

Dr. Kuhl, of West Germany, believes that all chronic diseases, including cancer, are caused by impaired cell-respiration and liver-damage. By this he means that the affected cells have been suffocated, choked with an excess of self-produced, pathologically-increased lactic acid. This excess of pathological lactic acid in the cell-fluid cannot be neutralized by taking chemicals, he says, because life does not follow the rules of chemistry. It can be removed, and cell-respiration regenerated, only by eating certain fermented foods, rich in *nutritional* lactic acid, because, strange as it may sound, the nutritional lactic acid in these foods drives out from the cell-fluid the stored pathologically-increased lactic acid which is impeding cell-respiration. Thus, cell-respiration can be regenerated. These fermented foods include fermented wheat-grains, fermented vegetable and plant juices, fermented milk-products (sour milk, cottage cheese, yoghourt, whey, etc.) and unleavened bread (obtainable on the Continent, but not in this country, although it *can* be made at home. It is simply bread-dough without yeast).

The fermented wheat-grains, and a lactic-acid plant-concentrate, also a recipe for making the unleavened bread (sourdough), can be obtained from Mr. E. L. David (Biological Research worker, 6 Redcliffe Close, Old Brompton Road, London, S.W.5). Or the fermented grains and the plant-concentrate can be made at home (much more cheaply) in a small apparatus he has designed for the purpose.

Fermented vegetable-juices, bottled in Switzerland, are now available in this country, and can be bought from most health-foods shops.

According to Dr. Jung of Germany, chronic degenerative diseases can be prevented by the daily consumption of 2–3 teaspoonfuls of *cold-pressed* vegetable oil, because it contains unsaturated fatty-acids.

It is an accepted fact that the body can combust animal fats (butter, cream, etc.) only when vegetable fats are also present. Both animal *and* vegetable fat, are, therefore, essential and equally important to the efficient functioning of the body and to good health. Vegetable fat acts as the spark which sets alight the fuel provided by animal fat. Vegetable fat is found in nuts of every kind, in nut butter, in vegetable-oil margarine, in soya-bean oil, sunflower seeds, sunflower-seed oil, safflower oil, linseed, sesame seeds, sesame-seed butter, corn oil, wheat-germ oil, etc. These are all obtainable from health-foods shops.

Cases of cancer are known to have recovered by fasting for a prolonged period (30–40 days) on vegetable-juices (chiefly carrot). The late Dr. Kirstin Nolfi of Denmark recovered from cancer of the breast in this way. When first she knew she had cancer, she lived for some weeks on raw kale juice, raw potato juice, raw carrot juice, and garlic. Thereafter, she lived exclusively on a raw fruit and vegetable diet for some years, and the cancer disappeared. She died many years later – and *not* from cancer. (Her very interesting little booklet, *The Raw-Food Treatment of Cancer and other Diseases* can be obtained from the London Vegetarian Society, 53 Marloes Road, London, W.8.)

Dr. Paul Kersch has also written a very helpful little book called *The Curability of Cancer* (The British Biochemic Association). He, too, believes that cancer can be caused by a shortage of potassium; that this can be remedied by daily doses of specially-prepared potassium-nitrate, and that the innate vitality of the body may then summon up all its power and produce a spontaneous cure. Such cures have been known to occur, he says.

Dr. Jules Samuels, M.D., of Amsterdam, believes that all degenerative diseases, including cancer, are chiefly caused by pituitary-gland imbalance. (The pituitary gland is the master-gland which controls all the other endocrine glands of the body.) His practice is to test all glands by means of a 'spectroscopic' blood-analysis; this reveals the faulty gland, and this he then treats with his special short-wave therapy, to increase or decrease (according to the result of the blood-analysis) its hormonal activity. He treats diabetes and disseminated sclerosis, as well as cancer.

To sum up the main points relating to the causes, prevention and treatment of cancer:

Its causes. These are thought to be:

1. Liver damage, due to wrong eating and drinking over a period of many years. By this is meant eating and drinking unnatural chemicalized foods; flesh foods; foods too hot or too cold, or too highly seasoned (because these foods are irritants to the lining of the digestive tract).

   Flesh foods are harmful not only because they are unclean and sometimes diseased, but because they give rise to bowel putrefactive toxins which poison the bloodstream. Also, they are growth-stimulants, and, as such, encourage our body cells (or some of them) to become rebels and grow too much.

2. A deficiency of catalase in the blood, caused by the presence of catalase-inhibiting substances in the air we breathe, in the foods we eat, in the water we drink, and the drugs and radiations with which we are medically treated; caused also by the eating of deficiency foods containing no catalase; and by a lack of outdoor exercise which stimulates the manufacture of catalase by our own bodies.

3. A lack of minerals in the blood, especially potassium, due to eating potassium-deficient foods grown on potassium-deficient soils, or to wrong and wasteful cooking-methods (e.g. discarding the vegetable cooking water); to the eating of too much common salt (which destroys potassium); to worry and other negative emotions which destroy potassium in our blood. The use of aluminium cooking-vessels is also detrimental, because aluminium, being an irritant, causes a loss of potassium.

4. A lack of oxygen in the blood, due to smog, smoke, and

fumes in the air we breathe; to lack of outdoor exercise; to oxygen-deficient water, and to badly-ventilated rooms, and to a lack of vitamin E, which off-sets loss of oxygen during fat-metabolism.

Prevention. Cancer could to a great extent be prevented by righting all the malpractices enumerated above; by educating people to understand and put into practice the basic principles of right eating and right cooking; by a drive, at international level, to improve soil conditions throughout the world by natural methods of fertilizing, and thus to improve food-production (not only the quantity but the quality of foods); by a campaign to encourage people to grow their own food (vegetables, fruits, cereals, etc.) and, as far as possible, to be self-supporting, fertilizing their crops with natural compost and animal wastes, rather than with fertilizers out of a packet which upset the chemical balance of the soil and destroy its population (earthworms, etc.).

Here is what Frank Wilson says on the subject of cancer, in *Food for the Golden Age* (The C. W. Daniel Co. Ltd., 60 Muswell Road, London, N.10).

It is not suggested that indulgence in animal foods is the only cause of cancer. In all probability cancer is a multiple disease, caused by many different unnatural things. Smoking and industrial chemicals in the air are undoubtedly connected with throat and lung cancers. But the growth-stimulating properties of animal foods are certainly among the most important and prevalent.

All the cells of our bodies start life in a semi-cancerous condition, tearing apart furiously in incessant division, but, as we grow older, substances are formed which quieten them down, and in the end just allow them to divide occasionally, to mend the small breaks and tears of life.

If, year in year out, we bombard these cells with substances which over-stimulate growth, some cells will one day break loose, for they must always be longing to leap back into their youthful freedom of promiscuous division – which is cancer.

Whatever stimulates our cells, thereby giving us a transient sense of well-being and making us possibly grow bigger, taller, and thicker, invites our cells to rebel. Cells are disciplined by Nature, and it may take years really to rouse them, but every little encouragement counts in the end.

The capacity of the body for healthfulness is truly immense, and many of the minor ills of life can be tackled without a call to a medico. Let us take advantage of a bout of disease to reform our way of living. And where the medico fails, especially in degenerative disease, there is always a chance of letting Nature have a go, though one cannot expect miracles. A disease like cancer is the result of long years of abuse, and the body's wisdom in 'curing' cancer is very limited, for cancer is a very new disease – a few hundred years are nothing in the history of our bodies – still, there is often a chance. But here again, if a cancer *is* diagnosed, for heaven's sake have it operated on and removed if it is not too late, and get any metastases treated by orthodox medical methods.

There is no question of doubt that they work in many cases, and not to make use of these aids and to rely on Nature in such a monstrously unnatural situation is to court certain death in many cases. With nature-cure, cancers *do* heal – at times – but one would have a much better chance if one had the cancer removed and *then* followed it up on the road to health with nature-cure and diet reform.

(Mr. Wilson's views about surgery are not shared by J. Ellis Barker, author of *Cancer, its Cause and Prevention*, and other eminent authorities.)

In the post-operational treatment of cancer, diet is very important, for, if the diet is not corrected and nutritional deficiencies not made good, it will recur. For full details of correct diet for cancer sufferers, see the books mentioned in 'Books for further reading' at the end of this book.

A grave dietetic error is the eating of too much salt. *Salt* (Sodium Chloride) is composed of sodium and chlorine (50 per cent of each). Sodium is an alkaline substance, chlorine is an acid. Both are essential to the human body. It is only when taken in excess of bodily requirements that salt becomes injurious and a danger to health. And it can so easily be taken in excess because so many of the foods we eat are already salted, to preserve them. For example, factory-made butter contains about 8 teaspoonfuls of salt to the pound ($\frac{1}{2}$ a teaspoonful to the ounce). Bakers use salt heavily in bread-making. Tinned meats, etc. contain salt; so do sausages, bacon, cheese, gravy flavourings, ice-cream and aspirin tablets. Most cooks add salt to vegetables to give them flavour, because vegetables lose their natural sodium (and other salts) in the cooking water. Meat contains sodium. Therefore, to add salt to meat, vegetables, and other foods, when we eat them, is to take it in excess, and to take it in excess is a danger to health. The explanation of why this is so is as follows:

The chlorine part of the salt we eat is seized by the stomach for the production of hydrochloric acid (an ingredient of the gastric juice which digests food in the stomach); the sodium part combines with carbon-dioxide (CO_2) gas (given off by body cells) to form carbonate of soda, a harmless substance which circulates in the blood so long as there is not an excess of it. If there *is* an excess of it, the excess breaks up into its components, CO_2 and Sodium (Na) and, in the absence of any acid with which to combine, the sodium component combines with water moisture, to form caustic soda (NaOH). This is a very powerful irritant, and, in order to protect themselves from it, the body cells start to multiply, because, when cells multiply, lactic acid is produced – the quicker they multiply, the more lactic acid is produced. The caustic soda is then able to combine with the lactic acid (alkaline substances tend to unite with acid substances and vice versa) and a harmless lactate-salt is formed, which is easily excreted from the body via the kidneys. So far, so good; it is when the body is in a debilitated state that the trouble begins, for it is then that the body cells are unable to produce sufficient lactic acid to neutralize, and combine with, the caustic soda; thus, the soda continues to irritate the cells, and the cells, in a frantic effort to produce enough lactic acid, continue to multiply, and a tumourous growth forms. If the irritation continues any length of time, the tumour may become cancerous. (A very helpful book on this subject is *Cancer, its Dietetic Cause and Cure* by Dr. Maud Fere, The Gateway Book Co., Gateway House, Bedford Park, Croydon, Surrey.)

Dr. Fere, who cured herself of cancer of the bowel, advises cancer sufferers to take doses of dilute hydrochloric acid. This will supplement the lactic acid which the cells are unable to produce in sufficient amounts to neutralize the caustic soda, and it will also supply the chlorine needed for the production of gastric juice.

She advises omitting all salt and salted foods from the diet, because, although sodium is necessary to the body, enough sodium will be obtained from meat, vegetables (especially celery and raw vegetables), salads (especially beetroot), and fruit (especially apples), making the addition of table-salt unnecessary and potentially dangerous.

Cancer of the breast and/or lung. A firm named Sandoz Ltd. of Basle in Switzerland, have produced an anti-cancer remedy from a species of the Podophyllum plant. It is obtainable only in Switzerland.

Cancer of the rectum. Iscador, the freshly-pressed juice of Viscum album (mistletoe) is used at the Rudolf Steiner Institute at Arlesheim in Switzerland. This remedy dates back to antiquity.

Cancer of the lymph glands, spleen, and liver, commonly called Hodgkin's disease. This has been successfully treated in America with an alkaloid, Vinchristine, derived from the Vinca Rosea (periwinkle) plant.

Cancer of the skin. Podophyllin, an extract from the plant Podophyllum, has been used with some success by Dr. Jonathan Hartwell of the National Cancer Institute, U.S.A.

Cancer of the blood (Leukaemia). Lymphocytic leukaemia in children is treated in the U.S.A. with Vinchristine, made from the Vinca Rosea plant. Granulocytic leukaemia is treated with an alkaloid related to Colchicine, which is derived from the Colchicum (Autumn Crocus) plant. Colchicine itself is a well-known remedy for gout.

It has been proved experimentally by Dr. Ferenczi of Hungary that raw beetroot juice has an inhibiting effect on cancerous growths, and on cancer of the blood. Professor Harris of the Microbiological Research Institute is experimenting with Folic acid (a B vitamin) to try to find bacteria that will destroy it, because it is a cell-growth stimulant.

Other natural anti-tumour remedies. These include anti-folic acid (a substance derived from yeast), extract of garlic, extract of bloodroot-herb, and raw beetroot juice. (See *Green Medicine* by Margaret Kreig, by Hodder and Stoughton, London.) Dried liver is remedial for its content of Resine, an anti-cancer substance.

Dr. Beard treats cancer with Chymotrypsin (see page 214, 'A Cancer Therapy'). Dr. Mary Catterall of the Medical Research Council uses Cyclotron treatment. Birkbeck College London are investigating natural chalones (substances in the blood that slow down cancer cell-division).

CATARRH

Not only are the nasal passages and the air passages connecting them with the lungs lined with a thin membrane called mucous membrane, but the vagina, the stomach, the intestines, the bile duct, and the colon are also lined with mucous membrane and liable, therefore, to become catarrhal.

Mucous membrane is so called because it secretes mucus, a transparent watery substance which not only lubricates the passages but sterilizes them. If mucous membrane is subjected to irritation, it becomes over-active and produces an abnormal amount of mucus, another name for which is catarrh. In the case of the air-passages (the nose, throat, windpipe, and bronchi) the irritation can be caused by fumes in the atmosphere (especially petrol fumes and cigarette smoke), by dust, by smog, and by chemicals used in (and on) foods. But by far the commonest cause, not only of nasal and bronchial catarrh but of vaginal, gastric, intestinal, and colonic catarrh, is systemic poisons circulating in the bloodstream. These poisons spring from an over-long retention, followed by a going-rotten process, of waste-products in the large bowel. They spring also from the fermentation and putrefaction that takes place in the large bowel when the wrong foods (or the wrong combination of even the *right* foods) are eaten.

By wrong foods is meant acid-producing, foodless foods, such as white bread and white-flour products, white sugar and white-sugar products, as well as the foods that, because they do not combine well together, are also acid-forming and clogging to the system. (See 'Compatible and Incompatible Foods'.)

Correct feeding is therefore all-important – as is also complete evacuation every day of all waste-products from the body, via the bowels, the kidneys, and the skin. To assist this, a dose of powdered compound of rhubarb should be taken at bed-time, once or twice a week, and ¼ teaspoonful of Glaubers salts in early-morning tea every day.

The quickest way to rid yourself of catarrh, which is Nature's attempt to rid the body of poisons, is first of all to fast for 2–3 days, taking only fresh (or dried) fruit, and liquids in the form of raw vegetable-juices, herb teas, etc. Alpine herb-tea is especially beneficial as it helps bowel action (see *Appendix*). Grapes and apples are better than citrus fruits. Dried fruits should include sun-dried Californian apricots (soaked overnight but not cooked); also Californian prunes, soaked overnight and simmered gently for half an hour, and, when cold, stoned, mashed, sweetened with molasses, and eaten with goat's milk yoghourt. Prune-juice (unsweetened) is obtainable (in tins) from health-foods shops, and a tablespoonful of this should be taken at intervals during the day. This will also help bowel action, but, to ensure thorough cleansing of the bowels, a purging dose of Epsom salts (a heaped teaspoonful in $\frac{1}{2}$ pint of hot water) should be taken first thing every morning, whilst fasting. If it does not thoroughly purge, double the dose next day, and again fast on juices only, for 24 hours.

After 2–3 days of fasting and of bowel-cleansing, the diet can be augmented by the addition of salads, cooked vegetables including potatoes cooked in their skins, cottage cheese, a little wholewheat bread, and an occasional egg, but flesh foods and cow's milk should be omitted. Granogen (soya-bean milk), dried skim-milk powder, plantmilk, and goat's milk yoghourt, should take the place of cow's milk, cream, and custard, etc. All starchy and sugary foods, such as cakes, biscuits, puddings, pies, pastry, sweets and chocolates, jams and jellies, etc. should also be avoided. Jellies are best made at home with fresh fruit-juices and 'Gelozone' (Irish Moss). Honey should replace sugar and sugar-products such as jams. Kelp powder (dried seaweed), garlic powder, and celery powder, should replace table-salt, though a little Bio-salt (Dr. Gilbert's) may be used, if desired.

Outdoor exercise every day is essential; walking, cycling, and horse-riding are all beneficial, especially walking if this is done with zest and enjoyment. Exercise should produce sweating and deepen the breathing. It should be followed by a warm bath or shower-bath, and a rub-down with a rough towel, to help elimination of waste-products through the skin, and to stimulate the production of body electricity.

Natural remedies include oil of garlic, and homoeopathic Hydrastis 30 (5 pilules night and morning).

Nasal catarrh (*chronic*). This is not in any way connected with the climate in which you live, i.e. with local weather conditions. Its cause, like that of all other kinds of catarrh, is usually faulty feeding habits, also lack of fresh air exercise. A cleansing and eliminative diet – preferably one that excludes all flesh foods, white bread and other white-flour products, white sugar, table-salt, and cow's milk, and that includes plenty of fresh fruit, salads and vegetables – would put an end to most people's catarrh, irrespective of where they live. Needless to say, if they reverted to the old bad habits of eating over-refined unnatural, and processed foods, it would return.

The orthodox medical treatment of chronic catarrh with suppressive drugs, sprays, drops, etc. is not only useless (because it does not tackle the underlying cause) but harmful; suppression of symptoms, which are Nature's external signs of internal disorder, is always wrong. However, a daily wash-out of the nostrils, using the juice of half a lemon in $\frac{1}{2}$ pint of warm water, does help, and, in addition to oil of garlic perles (3 a day), tincture of Hydrastis should be taken (5 drops in a teaspoonful of water, 3 times a day).

There are several homoeopathic remedies, including Rosemary 3x., Thuja 30, Kali. bichrom., or Sulph. 2x.

For chronic NASO – pharyngeal catarrh, the remedy is Eupatorium.

The biochemic remedy varies according to the colour and texture of the exuded catarrh. If it is a thick, white, sticky discharge, take Kali. mur. 6x., before meals. If it is of an albumenous nature, like uncooked white of egg, and semi-transparent, take Calc. phos. 6x., after meals. If it is thick, oily, and yellowish, take Kali. sulph. 6x., before meals.

Or take Dr. Gilbert's biochemic remedy. (See *Appendix*.)

A good herbal remedy for nasal and bronchial catarrh is

Antifect tablets, which contain garlic, echinacea, and veg. charcoal (see *Appendix*). Rosemary-herb tea is also helpful.

Bronchial catarrh. The advice given for nasal catarrh should be followed, avoiding starchy and sugary foods, using honey to sweeten drinks such as tea, and molasses in coffee. One of the best drinks for chest troubles of all kinds is linseed tea. (For recipe, see 'Herbal Recipes'.) Take sips whenever the catarrh causes coughing.

A homoeopathic remedy that loosens the catarrh is Eupatorium, 10–15 drops, 3 times a day.

For acute bronchitis take homoeopathic Ipecacuanha. 4x.

For bronchitis in T.B. people, the remedy is Myosotis Arvensis. 2x.

For chronic bronchitis a good remedy is Pinus sylvestris 2. (Stockholm tar).

Catarrh of the colon. See 'Colitis'.

Catarrh of the bladder. See 'Cystitis'.

Catarrh of eustachian tubes. Take Biochemic Kali. mur. 6x. before meals, Biochemic Calc. phos. 6x. after meals. Also 1 drop Tincture of Hydrastis 3 times daily.

Catarrh of the stomach. No food should be taken other than a small bowlful of 'Biobalm' food-beverage, to which a teaspoonful of acacia powder (gum-arabic) has been added, 4 times daily. Ideally, the Biobalm diet should be preceded by a short fast (24–48 hours), when nothing but sips of water and the undermentioned herbal and biochemic remedies should be taken. If the diet is strictly followed and no other foods eaten, the inflammation of the stomach should be healed in 7–10 days. The healing process can be helped by taking fluid extract of Golden Seal (Hydrastis) 3 times a day. The dose is 10 drops in a little hot water sipped slowly. After the first dose of the day, allow half a dozen pilules of biochemic Ferrum. phos. 6x. to dissolve slowly under the tongue. After the second dose, allow the same number of Nat. phos. pilules to dissolve in the mouth, and after the third dose take the same number of Kali. mur. pilules.

Catarrh of the vagina (Leucorrhea). The remedy depends upon the nature, colour and consistency of the exudation; a homoeopathic doctor should be consulted about this. Vaginal wash-outs, using 2 pints of warm water (previously boiled) to 10 drops of fluid extract of Hydrastis (Golden Seal) are cleansing, and will help to soothe and to allay irritation. Take either Hydrastis 3x. (2 pilules) before meals, and Ipecacuanha (2 pilules) after meals, or a cleansing internal remedy, such as a mixture of the following:

Fluid extract of Golden Seal (Hydrastis)	1 oz.
Tincture of Myrrh	1 oz.
Tincture of Echinacea	1 oz.

The dose is a small teaspoonful of the mixture in a little warm water, before meals.

CHANGE OF LIFE

This can be helped to pass more easily if a wineglassful of the following tea is taken once or twice a day:

Cover 1 oz. of motherwort herb and 1 oz. of tansy with 2 pints of water; bring to the boil, and simmer for 20 minutes. Strain, and sweeten to taste with honey. Calcium-lactate tablets are also a help. Small doses of sex hormones are prescribed by some doctors. They do help.

CHAPPED HANDS

Cover a slice of lemon with milk, leave for 2–3 hours, then use as a hand-cream.

CHEST COMPLAINTS

Bronchitis and asthma sufferers need extra vitamin A. They should take malt extract containing halibut liver oil; also vitamin E capsules (1 with meals). See 'Bronchitis'.

CHILBLAINS

These are usually a sign of lack of calcium in the blood; the remedy is to eat foods rich in calcium, such as yoghourt, cheese, soya-beans, almonds, millet seed, sesame seed, green vegetables, especially sprouts, kale, broccoli, and turnip tops. In addition, take 2 rose-hip and 2 Calcium-plus tablets with each meal; also 2 tablets of biochemic Silica every night at bedtime. Paint the chilblains with Friars Balsam (Tincture of Benzoin) if they are unbroken. If broken, use Marshmallow ointment or Tincture of myrrh. Take brisk outdoor exercise daily.

CHILDBIRTH (painless)

Start taking raspberry-leaf tea 2–3 times a week, 3 months before the birth is due. It should also be taken, hot, during labour, which it will help. Massage of the breasts with castor oil will also help labour, and will increase the milk-flow after the birth. Daily outdoor exercise (preferably walking) is essential. (See *Having a baby easily*, by Dr. M. Brady, Gateway Book Co.) If too great, the milk-flow can be reduced by drinking a tea made with periwinkle herb (Vinca major). Homoeopathia Nux Vomica is the remedy for morning sickness.

CHILDREN'S AILMENTS

These would fill a volume. They have been fully dealt with in *Baby and Child Care*, by Dr. Spock, in *Children's Health and Happiness*, by Dr. M. Brady (see Book-list, page 246).

For teething troubles there is no better remedy than Camomile tea, made strong, sweetened with honey, and given in teaspoonful doses.

One word of advice about vaccination against smallpox –

that word is 'don't'. The poisonous stuff used for a vaccination causes all kinds of health troubles in later life, if not immediately. The resulting troubles in later life, which include asthma, hay-fever, and skin troubles, are called 'vaccinosis' by Dr. Dorothy Shepherd, who deals with some of them in detail in her book *A Physician's Posy* (Health Science Press).

(See also *The Blood-poisoners*, by Lionel Dole, Gateway Book Co.)

CIRCULATORY DISTURBANCES

These include leg-ulcers, Buerger's disease, cardio-vascular disturbances, high blood-pressure, strokes, arteriosclerosis, heart-defects, anaemia due to lack of red blood-cells, cramps, pins and needles, giddiness, etc., all of which will be relieved if vitamin E (in the form of wheatgerm oil and vitamin E capsules) is taken regularly. This is because vitamin E prevents the formation in the blood of hydrogen-peroxide (a by-product produced when fats are oxidized), which destroys red blood-cells. A shortage of red blood-cells means that there will be a shortage of oxygen in the blood, because the red blood-cells are the carriers of oxygen, and this means that the tissues and organs of the body will not, therefore, receive sufficient oxygen, and will in consequence become disorganized or diseased. The liver and the heart, being the two organs that receive the largest quantity of blood, are the organs most affected by a deficiency of oxygen in the blood. Foods rich in vitamin E should therefore be eaten. These include sunflower (and other) seeds, nuts, wheatgerm, egg-yolk, soya-bean milk-powder, soya-bean oil, watercress, lettuce, etc.

Deficiency of oxygen in the blood can also be remedied by inhalation of a substance made from the rare element Cerium, called Lanthasol. This substance is sprayed out, by a machine called a nebulizer, in the form of a very fine spray. The patient sits in front of the machine and inhales the fine spray, but only 4–5 times on the first day. The inhalations are repeated daily for several weeks, the number being increased each day. The tiny droplets of the inhaled Lanthasol penetrate to the alveoli of the lungs, and from there into the bloodstream. Here they ensure that the oxygen in the blood is transported to all the cells of the body, and is fully utilized.

Respiratory diseases are also greatly benefited by this treatment, as there is always a shortage of oxygen in the blood of people with chest complaints, such as asthma, emphysema, chronic bronchitis, etc. The treatment is available in Germany but not in England. (For further details, see *Some Adventures in Healing*, by Dr. Graupner.)

COELIAC DISEASE

This is a children's disease, the cause of which is unknown. The symptoms are loss of appetite (with consequent malnutrition and wasting of body-tissues), diarrhoea, and sometimes vomiting of food. The answer to the feeding problem of such children is ripe bananas, mashed up together with a little whey powder, a teaspoonful of carob-bean powder, a little boiled water, and some skim-milk powder.

Bananas contain protein and vitamin C. They are liked and accepted by most children with coeliac disease, whereas quite often these children will not accept the usual prepared infant-foods; nor should they be given wheat or oats in any form, as these contain 'gluten', which is harmful to, and not tolerated by, them. A list of gluten-free foods can be obtained from the Secretary of the Coeliac Society, 116 London Road, London, N.W.8. Gluten-free flour called wheat starch, and gluten-free baking powder, for home bread-making, can be obtained from Energen Foods Ltd., Pound Lane, Willesden, London N.W. 10.

At first, the diet should be confined to mashed bananas, skim-milk, and fruit juices, but gradually, as absorption improves as a result of the gluten-free diet, other foods can be added to the diet, such as Casilan (milk-protein), lightly boiled egg-yolk, junket, jelly made with fruit juice and Gelozone, and a little bread and butter.

Most children recover slowly but completely.

THE COMMON COLD

It is a mistake to take things to suppress a cold, which is Nature's way of forcing you to rest, so that your body can throw out unwanted debris that has accumulated in the blood. An unclean bloodstream, loaded with unwanted debris, provides a favourable breeding-ground for the common-cold virus, which cannot live and multiply in a clean bloodstream because it requires waste-matter on which to feed. It gains entry into the body via the nose or mouth, but, if waste-matter is not present in the blood, it will have nothing to feed on and will soon die and be excreted, together with other unwanted debris, through the eliminative organs of the body. A clean bloodstream is, therefore, the best insurance against all forms of germs, including the cold-virus and the 'flu-virus.

The feverish condition of the blood, which usually accompanies a cold or 'flu, provides the bonfire, so to speak, for the burning-up of the debris. It is a mistake, therefore, to suppress it – to try to put out the fire – by taking drugs such as aspirin (though sometimes a little dose of bicarbonate of soda or a piece of raw onion held in the mouth for a few hours, will scotch an oncoming cold). The thing to do is to rest as much as possible (preferably in bed, where you are warmest) and to abstain from eating solid food for 24–48 hours. Hot lemonade with a pinch of cinnamon and a little honey in it, and hot elderflower-and-mint tea, with a pinch of composition powder in it, will induce sweating and excretion of waste-products through the skin. The body should be rubbed down with a rough towel; this will remove the sweat, and will induce further sweating and further elimination of unwanted debris through the pores of the skin. If there is no rise in temperature, a warm bath may be taken, using a bath-brush to friction the skin and, if you can go straight to bed after it, half a pound of common Epsom salts should be added to the water. At bedtime, take a teaspoonful dose of laxative herbs, such as Innerclean, with a drink of hot lemonade, or a cup of Alpine-herb tea, or a dose of compound (powdered) rhubarb. This should ensure a good bowel movement, but to make doubly sure of a thorough bowel cleansing, take 1 teaspoonful of Epsom salts in $\frac{1}{2}$ pint of hot water, next morning, followed by a hot drink (tea, or whatever you fancy), but again, no solid food for 24 hours – just hot drinks, and fruit juices. In between the drinks, suck acerola tablets. These are rich in vitamin C, which is a powerful (natural) antibiotic and germ-killer. Eucalyptus is also a powerful germ-killer. As well as inhaling it, it can be taken internally – 2 drops in a small teaspoonful of honey, with a mouthful of hot liquid, 2–3 times a day.

If the nose and throat are very congested, and the head feels bloated and heavy, a hot foot-bath with a tablespoonful of mustard in it will help to decongest it. For the head, place a cold wet compress (or pad) on the forehead and bridge of the nose, and for the throat, a cold wet bandage round the throat; this can be secured in place by tying an old stocking over it. A cold wet bandage, about 8–9 inches wide, round the waist, covered with a wider piece of flannel, can be applied at night, removed in the morning, and washed thoroughly.

Inhalations of steaming water, impregnated with 2 drops of eucalyptus oil, or $\frac{1}{2}$ teaspoonful of Friars Balsam, or a crystal of Menthol, will relieve congestion of the throat and chest. A suitable container is a 'Dr. Nelson' inhalation jar, made of earthenware. Everyone who suffers with chronic chest colds and bronchial troubles should use one, and should take Dr. Gilbert's biochemic specific remedy for colds and bronchitis (see *Appendix*).

After 2 days on hot drinks and juices, fruit may be eaten – oranges, grapes, apples, and bananas (mashed up) with yog-hourt; also raw vegetable-juices (obtainable, in bottles, from health-foods shops; the elderflower-and-mint remedy is also obtainable, ready for use).

On the third or fourth day, the cold should have subsided and a more normal diet can be taken, although to live entirely on fruit for a whole week can do nothing but good; it cleanses the entire system. (See *How to banish colds and influenza*, by George Hall, N.D. (Gateway Book Co.).

COLITIS

This is inflammation of the colon (large intestine). There are two kinds of colitis, mucous and ulcerative. Both are the result of prolonged irritation of the delicate membrane which lines the walls of the colon. The irritation *can* be due to chronic constipation, and to the taking of purgatives for the constipation. The constipation causes an accumulation on the walls of the colon of hard faecal matter, which is never properly evacuated, and the purgatives (which do not remove the accumulation) simply increase the irritation. Warm water wash-outs are the only way of softening and of removing these accumulations of hardened matter with which the walls of the colon have become encrusted. Plain warm water (previously boiled) should be used to which 1 teaspoonful of pure olive oil has been added. They should be given daily for the first few days, but discontinued as soon as the bowels start to function normally. The inflammation can also be caused by 'auto-immunity'. (See 'Ulcerative colitis'.)

The orthodox treatment of colitis with bowel wash-outs containing suppressive drugs is based upon the assumption that colitis is due to germ infection. This is not so. The suppressive drugs cause a driving-back into the system of the toxic matter in the colon which Nature is trying to eliminate in the form of mucus. They (the drugs) suppress the symptoms for a time, but they do nothing to remove the *cause* of the symptoms, which will, therefore, recur, and the colitis will become chronic. Bowel wash-outs with suppressive drugs do no good and *may* do harm. Bowel wash-outs *are* necessary, as already stated, but only plain water (or plain water with a little olive oil) should be used.

The correction of the diet is of primary importance. For the first 2–7 days (depending upon the severity of the trouble), nothing but raw apples, yoghourt, raw vegetable-juices, and Slippery-elm food-beverage, should be taken. (These can be taken alternately every 2 hours.) The juices should be diluted with a little boiled water. Lemon juice, celery juice, carrot juice, and raw apples, are especially beneficial.

After about 1 week on the semi-fasting diet, malted-milk, also whey powder sprinkled on finely-ground wheatgerm cereal, may be added to the diet. ('Viga-Vyte' is an extra-fine wheatgerm.) Mashed-up ripe banana with goat's milk yoghourt, or plantmilk, also pulped or grated raw apple mixed with 1 teaspoonful of apple-pectin, are soothing to the inflamed membranes, and may now be eaten. Apple-pectin eaten with raw pulped apples is a most valuable remedy for colitis; a trickle of honey may be eaten with it, if liked. Pectin is obtainable from most good chemists.

The late Dr. Dudley Wright, eminent physician and surgeon, advised colitis sufferers to ingest nothing but raw pulped (or grated) apples and plenty of water (previously boiled), on 2 consecutive days, every week, for several months. As many as 20 apples per day (with added pectin) could be eaten, he said, but they must be raw, and of course really ripe. On the other days, a teacupful of a decoction made of stewed linseed, wheat-bran, and cut-up potatoes (unpeeled), should be eaten with raw carrot-juice, every 2 hours. The decoction should be sieved before the carrot-juice is added. A 5-drop dose of the fluid-extract of Agrimony-herb should be taken 3 times a day, together with $\frac{1}{4}$ teaspoonful of Composition powder.

After about 2 weeks on the above diet, the symptoms should have eased considerably, but, if they have not eased, you must continue with it a little longer. As soon as they do ease, the following foods, rich in vitamin B, should be added: wholewheat bread (toasted, and well-masticated), 1–4 teaspoonfuls of Yestamin powder (brewer's yeast) on fine wheatgerm cereal, and either minced liver or dried-liver tablets. (If you are a vegetarian, a B.12 tablet daily can replace liver.) Other things that can gradually be added to the diet, provided they do not aggravate the symptoms, are potatoes (cooked in their jackets, then peeled and mashed), a lightly-boiled egg, and a clear vegetable soup made with potato-water, lentils, linseed, onions, carrots, leeks, and brown barley. A teaspoonful of soya-bean oil may be used on the mashed potatoes, and a little unsalted butter on the toast.

Things that should be excluded from the diet are white sugar, white bread and white-flour products, highly seasoned foods, salted foods, foods cooked in aluminium pans, unboiled water, and strong tea.

A vegetarian diet is preferable to one in which flesh foods are included; cheese, eggs, soya-bean, Casilan (dried milk) take the place of flesh foods, are far more digestible and, therefore, less clogging to the system. (Cheese should be finely grated.)

Salt should be replaced by garlic powder, which can be used liberally. Dandelion coffee should replace ordinary coffee.

The main items of diet should, therefore, be clear vegetable soups, raw vegetable juices, potatoes cooked in their jackets (mashed), conservatively-cooked carrots and green vegetables (mashed), cheese (grated), egg dishes, wheatgerm, malted milk, Slippery-elm food-beverage, mashed raw apples and bananas, goat's-milk yoghourt, plant-milk, soya-bean milk and Casilan. 'Florus' powder should be taken night and morning (see *Appendix*). This encourages the growth of beneficial bacteria (the normal inhabitants of the large bowel) and discourages the growth of harmful bacteria.

Ulcerative colitis. This very serious ailment *can* be the result of what is known in the medical world as 'Auto-

Immunity'. This is an abnormal reaction of the body to one of its own tissues – a rejection of the tissue, which it regards as an intruder; in colitis it is the lining of the colon that is regarded as an intruder and disowned. The mistake the body makes in regarding its own tissue thus is due to a breakdown in its 'tolerance mechanism', and this breakdown is thought to be due to deep-seated emotional causes within the subconscious mind. To get rid of these subconscious emotions, they must be brought up to the level of the conscious mind, faced up to, and discussed with an understanding person, possibly a doctor with a knowledge of psychoanalysis. It is thought that auto-immunity *could* be caused by a deep-seated dislike of self, and that the body will continue to treat its own tissue as an intruding foreign substance so long as it continues to dislike itself. The 'tolerance mechanism' can be righted only by a conscious facing-up to the guilt-sense that is causing the dislike of self and the consequent calling-up of the body's militia (the antibodies that are fighting and destroying the body's own tissue). Once the dislike of self has been removed, the 'tolerance mechanism' will right itself, the damage will stop, and the affected part (in this case, the colon) will regain normality. Research into ways of suppressing the 'auto-immunity' process ('auto-allergy' would be a better name for it) – of curing it – goes hand in hand with research into ways of suppressing tissue-rejection of transplanted organs; it is not yet understood how or why either process occurs, though in the case of transplanted organs, which *are* foreign intruders, it is more understandable.

The fight that takes place between the body's militia and an invading germ destroys not only the germ but the surrounding tissue, causing damage and sometimes haemhorrage. But this fight is short-lived and the damage only temporary, unlike the fight that takes place between the body's militia and its own tissues; *this* fight may become prolonged and do much damage unless it is terminated by a return to normal of the 'tolerance-mechanism'.

The diet for ulcerative colitis should be much the same as

for mucous colitis, except that it should exclude all roughage for a time, until the symptoms subside. This means that no rough bread should be eaten, that fruit should be peeled, vegetables mashed. The perfect food is mashed banana. Colitis has been fully dealt with in *Encyclopaedia of Digestive Disorders*, by Frank Roberts, M.N.I.M.H. (Thorsons Ltd).

CONSTIPATION

This is not a disease, and can be cured by natural methods, but, although not a disease, it is the pre-disposing cause of many diseases, including arthritis, appendicitis, colitis, cancer, high blood-pressure, etc. It is also the cause of many minor ailments such as tiredness, headaches, inability to concentrate, etc.

Constipation is the over-long retention in the bowel of a large accumulation of waste matter (mostly food-residues after all the nutrients have been extracted from the food). This putrefies (goes rotten) if not excreted regularly every 24 hours, the resulting putrefactive toxins and gases being re-absorbed into the system and causing auto-intoxication (self-poisoning). Flesh foods are especially liable to cause putrefaction in the bowel, and a fleshless diet is preferable for this reason (and for many other reasons). If flesh foods *are* eaten, a cupful or two of yoghourt should be a regular daily item of diet, because yoghourt encourages the growth of beneficial bacteria in the bowel, and discourages the growth of putrefactive bacteria.

Constipation can be due to any one (or more) of the following causes:

1. A diet of over-refined, de-natured, unnaturally-concentrated food, robbed of its 'roughage'. White bread and other white-flour products, white sugar and white-sugar products, meat, boiled vegetables – these things are sadly deficient in natural roughage, which has been removed from them, and in minerals, vitamins, and digestive en-

zymes, which have been destroyed in the cooking of them. They are, therefore, unbalanced foods. Natural foods are balanced foods, that is to say, they retain all their parts, including their roughage, i.e. their skins, in the case of vegetables and fruits, and the bran (outer husk) and germ, in the case of cereals (wheat, etc.).

Roughage is not absorbed by the body, but it is an essential part of our diet, because, after the food-nutrients have been absorbed into the blood, it is the part that stimulates the rhythmic contractions of the bowel (known as peristalsis). These contractions push all residual wastes towards the bowel-exit (the rectum). If there were no roughage in the bowel, the bowel muscles would have nothing to grasp or to push against, and they would become flabby and lazy. This is exactly what *does* happen in many cases of constipation, when it is caused by a lack of roughage in the diet.

2. Another cause of constipation is the habit of eating over-refined cooked foods. These take up less space in our insides than do natural raw foods; the consequence is that most people over-eat, over-loading their digestive systems with highly-concentrated, devitalized foods of all kinds (mostly cooked), which simply clog the body-mechanism without giving it the vital thing it needs for its sustenance and repair-work. It is impossible to over-eat if we eat only natural (mostly uncooked) foods, because these are bulky; the consequence is, we are able to eat less of them, and yet they provide us with everything we need, including vitamins, minerals, and roughage.

Cooking destroys the ferments and vitamins in flesh foods; these are essential for its proper digestion and absorption; so, since it cannot be eaten raw, it is better omitted from the diet and replaced by cheese, eggs, nuts and seeds, soya beans, lentils, etc. These are better sources of protein than flesh foods, for the simple reason that they can be completely digested and absorbed; cooked flesh foods cannot.

3. Another cause of constipation can be nervous debility, due to worry, over-work, late hours, etc. Nervous debility causes continuous tension of the bowel muscles, and this causes spastic constipation. For this, Lactose (milk-sugar) in the form of powdered whey (or lacto-flora tablets) should be taken with food, and 1 tablespoonful of Florus powder taken in a little milk twice a day, half an hour before meals. Foods rich in calcium, such as yoghourt, hard (not soft) cheese, and foods rich in potassium, such as spinach and other green vegetables that have been organically grown on mineral-rich soil, should be eaten; also carrots. They are best eaten raw (juiced in a juice-press). If cooked, their minerals get lost in the cooking-water and thrown away. Salt robs the body of potassium. It should be replaced by kelp (powdered seaweed) and garlic powder.

Anaemia is often another cause of constipation, because it causes flabbiness of all the muscles of the body, including the bowel muscles. (See 'Anaemia'.)

The continuous use of laxatives and purgatives causes constipation, because they act as a whip acts on a tired horse; they produce a momentary spurt, followed by a greater tiredness and an inability to work at all without them. Thus, as time goes on, they have to be increased in size and strength. Liquid paraffin, although not a drug, is a mineral oil, and passes through the body without being absorbed, but, in its passage through the body, it carries with it the fat-soluble vitamins A, D, and E, thus robbing the body of these important vitamins. Anyway, none of these things (laxatives, purgatives, paraffin, etc.) will be needed if the diet is corrected, if outdoor exercise with deep breathing is taken every day, and if plenty of fresh vegetables, vegetable-juices, and fresh and sun-dried fruits are eaten. Apples are especially valuable; also dates, prunes, and figs.

Bedridden people who are unable to take outdoor exercise should be shown by a physiotherapist how to do exercises in bed, and should be given abdominal massage and limb massage.

Treatment. The whole of the digestive tract should be given a complete rest from solid food for a few days (only fruit or raw vegetable juices taken) and a thorough cleansing by taking 'Innerfresh' tablets with a drink of water, every night at bedtime, for a week. These mild herbal tablets will stimulate the mucous lining of the bowel to secrete mucus which will remove old hardened encrustations adhering to the bowel wall. Bowel wash-outs (with a 'gravity' douche) once or twice a week are also advisable; these *can* be self-given, but they are best administered by an expert physiotherapist at some naturopathic establishment, where expert medical supervision and advice, also correct diet, is obtainable. It is difficult to treat oneself properly at home; there is always the temptation to eat when you see other people eating. There is no such temptation when staying at a curative establishment where some of the other people round you are also fasting, where delicious drinks are prepared for you every few hours, and where a bowel wash-out is so expertly done that it is not an ordeal. Chiropractic treatment, which eases pressure on intestinal nerves, thus enabling the bowel to evacuate more freely, is also obtainable at a naturopathic establishment. (See *Appendix*.)

During the few days of fasting and of bowel wash-outs you may not feel too good; this is because your body is trying to rid itself of effete matter and toxic substances. Take things easy, but there is no need to stay in bed all day; in fact, it is better to take some outdoor exercise, so long as you stop short of over-tiredness.

After the few days of fasting on raw juices, the diet for the next week to 10 days should consist of fresh fruit, vegetables, raw vegetable-juices, and yoghourt (yoghourt is obtainable at health-foods shops), and then salads, grated cheese, wholewheat bread and a little unsalted butter can be added, so that at the end of about 3 weeks, 2 meals a day are being eaten, based on the following lines:

On rising. A glassful of hot water containing the juice of half a lemon. A little honey may be added. (Honey is a laxative.)

Breakfast. Prunes (soaked overnight in water to which 1 teaspoonful of molasses has been added), together with 1 tablespoonful of All-bran, 1 teaspoonful of powdered agar-agar, and ½ cupful of yoghourt, make a good laxative breakfast. The prunes, if well soaked, will not need cooking; sun-dried apricots can be soaked in the same way, and eaten instead of the prunes sometimes. A cup of dandelion coffee, sweetened with molasses, can be taken; also toast and butter.

Lunch at midday. (Interchangeable with the evening meal.) This should consist of a plateful of ground-up raw grains (wheat, barley, and groats), ground-up seeds (sunflower, pumpkin, sesame, buckwheat, millet, and linseed), a few ground-up nuts, 1 tablespoonful of wheatgerm, 1 tablespoonful of whey powder, Malvern water to moisten, and some diluted plantmilk. The raw grains should be ground up the night before, placed in a porridge or soup plate, covered with 2 tablespoonfuls of boiling water, and left to soak all night. This softens them quite sufficiently to make them digestible. Next morning, add the ground-up seeds, etc. This meal should be thoroughly chewed, eaten slowly, and not accompanied or followed by any liquid.

Afternoon tea. A pot of tea in which a teaspoonful of Potter's Alpine-herb is blended with ordinary tea. This is slightly laxative, and has a pleasant taste. Sweeten with honey, not sugar.

Evening meal. This should include a mixed raw salad of lettuce, cress, tomato, radishes, grated carrot, beetroot, etc., dressed with sunflower-seed oil, wholewheat bread (toasted), a baked potato in its skin, farmhouse or cottage cheese, or an egg-and-cheese savoury. It should be preceded by a wine-glassful of raw vegetable juices (mixed), prepared just before needed. (Never prepare it hours in advance, because this means loss of vitamins.) Bottled vegetable juices (carrot, celery, beetroot, and tomato) can be bought at most health-foods shops. A cup of dandelion coffee sweetened with black molasses, and a few dates or figs or raisins, may follow this meal, but no acid fruits should be eaten with it. An apple or apple-juice may be taken at bedtime; it will help to ensure sound sleep.

Especially important is daily exercise in the fresh air; a short brisk walk, accompanied by deep breathing as you stride along, is one of the best form of exercise. A few minutes should also be spent every day in doing body-bending and trunk-rolling exercises. These stimulate the liver to produce bile, which assists bowel-movement.

A bi-weekly dose of powdered rhubarb compound ($\frac{1}{2}$ tea-spoonful) should be taken at bedtime. It can be mixed with, and its taste disguised by, a little honey. An alternative laxative is Alexandrian senna pods (10 pods soaked in water for 8 hours, taken at bedtime). An added pinch of ginger will prevent any griping pains. A nightly dose (1 teaspoonful) of Psyllum seeds or of 'Agiolax' will provide 'bulk' (see *Appendix*).

CORNS AND CALLOUSES

At bedtime, soak the feet in a bowl of warm water, to which a small handful of common Epsom salts has been added; then massage the feet with castor oil. Sleep in loose cotton socks, to keep the oil off the sheets. When available, a strip of pineapple peel bandaged on to a corn will cure it. When not available, use a piece of lint soaked in oil of turpentine, or paint with a proprietary 'corn-cure', every day for a week.

CORONARY THROMBOSIS

Animal fats (saturated fatty-acids) should be replaced almost entirely by vegetable-oil fats (unsaturated fatty-acids). However, owing to their 'unsaturated' nature, their molecules easily attach to oxygen with which they combine to form hydrogen-peroxide, a rancid substance which poisons the bloodstream. Their attachment to oxygen causes a shortage of oxygen in the blood, and this calls for the production of more red blood-cells, carriers of oxygen. But an increase of red blood-cells (resulting from a lack of oxygen in the blood) thickens the blood (increases its viscosity). If the blood-viscosity is high, the circulation is slowed and there is increased strain on the heart, leading to heart attacks.

So, in order to prevent the lack of oxygen in the blood, caused by the intake of unsaturated fatty-acids contained in vegetable oils, some vitamin E should be taken every day (with food). Vitamin E prevents the oxidation of these oils; it ensures that oxygen is not wasted in this way, and that the blood has an adequate oxygen supply without an over-production of red blood-cells, which tend to thicken it and to make it less free-flowing.

All vegetable oils (if they have been 'cold-pressed' and not heat-treated) contain lecithin and E.F.A. (Essential Fatty Acids), safflower oil and soya-bean oil being especially rich in them. Lecithin is an homogenizer – that is to say, it breaks up fat and cholesterol into tiny particles, thus preventing them from adhering to the walls of the arteries and causing blockages. Foods that contain lecithin are egg-yolk, *un*pasteurized raw milk, soya-beans, sesame seeds, sunflower seeds, millet seeds, corn-kernels, wheatgerm, nuts, whole rice, whole barley, whole wheat, groats (dehusked oats) etc. Vegetable oils (so long as they are obtained by the 'cold-pressed' method of extraction and not by heat-treatment), are very rich in lecithin, vitamins E and B, and Essential Fatty Acids. But, if they are obtained by the heat-treatment

101

method, or if they are 'hydrogenated' (i.e. if hydrogen is added to them, to harden and whiten them and make them easier to handle when pastry-making, cake-making or frying), their vitamins, lecithin, and E.F.A. are destroyed in the process. So, do not eat any fats that have been tampered with (i.e. hydrogenated), nor margarine. This, although made from vegetable oils, has been heat-treated, so that no vitamins or lecithin remain in it. Use instead cold-pressed vegetable oil (wheatgerm or safflower) which is obtainable from health-foods shops.

COUGHS

Coughs can be relieved by drinks of linseed and liquorice tea, which is made as follows: Cover 1 oz. whole linseed, 1 oz. wild thyme, and ½ oz. of horehound herb with 2½ pints of boiling water. Stir, and allow to stand in a warm place for ½ hour. Strain into a jug, adding 1 oz. of liquorice extract, the juice of a lemon, and 1 tablespoonful of honey. (The linseed should be whole seed, not the crushed sort used for poultices.) Take sips of the tea when the cough is troublesome.

Rub the chest and back with warmed camphorated oil, or Olbas oil (see *Appendix*).

A homoeopathic remedy for a troublesome cough is Lungwort, or a herb-tea can be made of Lungwort herb.

CRAMP

This is very often due to a calcium deficiency, so the remedy is to step-up your intake of calcium-rich foods, especially yoghourt made of goat's milk (obtainable from many health-foods shops), and to take 'Calcium-Plus' tablets. To ensure their absorption, a teaspoonful of cider-vinegar in a little water should be taken with them, at meal-times. To provide fatty-acids also necessary for the absorption of the calcium a little vegetable oil should be eaten on salads. Extra vitamin C, in the form of rose-hip or acerola tablets, is also necessary for absorption of calcium.

Table-salt should be replaced by kelp powder or Bio-salt (Dr. Gilbert's), both of which contain potasssium and iodine, which also help calcium-absorption. Manual workers who sweat profusely, lose a lot of salt, and this (a lack of sodium chloride in the blood) can cause cramp, so these people should use Bio-Salt, as well as kelp.

CYSTITIS

See 'Bladder troubles'.

DEBILITY

Three important vitamins of the B complex, vitamin B.1 (thiamine), vitamin B.12 (cobalamine) and folic acid, should be taken with the daily diet (see 'Anaemia'). Vitamin C intake should also be stepped up (rose-hips, blackcurrants, and citrus fruits are rich in vitamin C). Liver (dried and powdered or in tablet form) is rich in all the B vitamins. A good herbal tea to take is made as follows: Simmer together in 2 pints of water for about $\frac{1}{2}$ hour (in a lidded saucepan) 1 tablespoonful of Camomile herb and garden sage, 6 tablespoonfuls of wheat-bran, 1 teaspoonful of gentian root (powdered), and 1 tablespoonful of wild marjoram herb. Then add 1 tablespoonful of buchu leaves, allow them to infuse for a few minutes, stir well, allow to cool with the lid on, then add 1 tablespoonful of wild thyme. Allow to stand for several hours, then strain and bottle. Keep in a cool place, and take a wineglassful before meals. A trickle of honey can be added to make it palatable.

A good homoeopathic remedy is Arnica 30. Take 4 pilules dry on the tongue at bedtime and before breakfast for several weeks.

A diet high in calories does *not* create energy. It actually decreases it. Body energy is a form of neuro-electricity produced in the cells of the brain. It is the result of the chemical reaction involved in the oxidation of food-nutrients in the brain-cells. The electrical charge thus created is a very minute one, but when it is combined with the charges from other brain-cells, it is sufficient to produce a flow of nervous energy – a nervous impulse – to whatever part of the body one desires to influence. Correct nutrition of the body is therefore all-important to the functional integrity of the body – i.e. to its ability to function energetically – and most important in a nutritionally-correct diet are the mineral-salts and trace-elements, without which all other nutrients are useless for body-building, body-maintenance, and energy-production. If these are missing from the diet, food nutrients are useless, the production of nervous energy ceases, and slowly the body dies. (For good sources of mineral-salts and trace-elements, see my *Handbook of Health,* Thorsons Ltd.)

DERMATITIS

This can sometimes be due to a lack of E.F.A. (Essential Fatty Acids) in the diet, and so can often be cured by adding a spoonful or two of vegetable oil (cold-pressed soya-bean oil, or sunflower-seed oil, or corn oil) to the diet.

DIABETES

This is the result of a deficiency of a substance called Insulin produced by the pancreas. The deficiency is often due not so much to a breakdown in the ability of the pancreas to produce sufficient insulin as to the inability of the insulin to do its job properly, owing to blood-impurity or to opposition. Blood impurity is caused by incorrect feeding. The opposition can come from various sources; for example, from the body's 'anti-bodies' (its defence corps) which combine with the insulin and neutralize it; from the liver cells, which can imprison it; from pituitary-gland, adrenal-gland, thyroid-gland, or even the pancreas itself, some of whose hormones may oppose the action of insulin and prevent it from doing its job properly. The interference by these gland hormones is being investigated by present-day research. It is treated with short-wave therapy by Dr. Samuels of Amsterdam (see page 193).

A thorough internal cleansing, combined with diet-reform, are two of the most important remedial measures. A warm water bowel wash-out should be given every day for a few days, plus a nightly dose of tincture of rhubarb. If insulin is being taken, the diabetic should not fast; he should simply reform his daily diet, eliminating flesh-foods, starches, and sugars of all kinds, and living for the first week or so on raw fruit, raw vegetables and salads, raw vegetable-juices, and goat's milk yoghourt. Beans *and* their pods *and* the water in which they are cooked should be eaten. As soon as tests show that the sugar-content of the urine is getting less (which it will do if the diet is corrected, if the bowels are working freely, and if the bean-pod water is being drunk every day) the doses of insulin can be reduced.

Bean pods contain an insulin-like substance which contains silicic acid. This is of great medicinal value not only to diabetics but also to arthritics. The water in which the beans and their pods are cooked should be taken, in small amounts, between meals. When the beans are out of season and unavailable, homoeopathic Phaseolus pilules (derived from the beans) should be taken. The dose is 5 pilules night and morning.

Garlic helps to reduce the sugar-content of the urine. It should be taken as part of the daily diet. Garlic perles are tasteless and odourless; they should be taken with meals. Garlic powder should be used instead of salt.

It is erroneously thought that a diabetic should not take raw juice of root vegetables because they mostly contain sugar. But this sugar is natural sugar and is quite different from the refined sugar sold in food-shops. It is actually beneficial to diabetics; so, too, are the juices of ripe citrus fruits (oranges, lemons, grapefruit, etc.). However, bananas, also sugar-containing fruits such as dates, raisins, sultanas, etc. should be avoided at first. Later, when the sugar-content of the urine has decreased, they too can be eaten.

Other important foods that diabetics should eat include cucumber, watercress, celery, celeriac, artichokes, garlic, leeks, and onions. The juice of cucumber contains an enzyme which stimulates the cells of the pancreas to produce insulin. Cucumber should be eaten (or juiced) with the peel on. It should be eaten every day when obtainable, together with other salad greens, including dandelion leaves, watercress, little onions, radishes, garlic, lettuce, parsley, etc. When not obtainable, dehydrated juice of cucumber, watercress, garlic, nettles, etc. can be obtained, in powder form. (See 'Juices', in *Appendix*.)

Condiments and table-salt should be replaced by kelp powder, garlic powder, celery powder, and onion powder. If salt *is* used, it should be Bio-salt. Salad-dressing should be made of cider-vinegar and sunflower-seed oil, mixed in equal parts.

Animal fats, including butter, should be replaced to a great extent by vegetable fats and oils, including soya-bean oil, sunflower-seed oil and sunflower-seed oil margarine. Nothing but vegetable oil should be used for cooking. Animal fats produce cholesterol deposits in the blood-vessels, which may shut off the circulation to the legs so completely that gangrene of the toes or feet may occur. Also, oxidation of animal-fats produces hydrogen-peroxide, which destroys red blood-cells (the carriers of iron), hence, the blood of diabetics who eat animal-fats is usually deficient in iron as well as oxygen. For these reasons, the consumption of animal-fats should be reduced to about $\frac{1}{2}$ oz. per day.

Dandelion coffee should replace ordinary coffee, and tea made with vinca-rosea herb should partly replace ordinary tea (see *Appendix*). Half a teacupful twice a day is enough. It is as efficacious as insulin.

As soon as sugar in the urine diminishes, a little home-made potato-bread may be included in the diet, but not more than about 2 oz. a day. It should be made of soya flour, mashed-up cold potatoes that have been boiled in their skins then peeled, and wholewheat flour, in equal amounts.

Oats and oatmeal are very valuable foods for diabetics. They contain an insulin-like substance called saponin. A teaspoonful of dehusked oats (groats) or 1 tablespoonful of oatflakes, should be ground-up in a coffee-mill and soaked in a little boiling water for 10 minutes. To this add 1 tablespoonful of wheatgerm, a little milk to moisten, a sprinkling of Yestamin (brewer's yeast powder) and 1 vitamin B.12 tablet (see *Appendix*), this 'muesli' to be eaten at least once a day. It can, to some extent, take the place of bread.

Outdoor exercise, combined with deep breathing, is of great importance to diabetics, because their blood is usually deficient in oxygen. Daily rubbing of the whole body with vinegar is beneficial.

As already mentioned, Dr. Jules Samuels of Amsterdam successfully treats diabetes with his short-wave therapy. This treatment stimulates the pancreas to produce its own insulin, and does away with the necessity for insulin injections. The treatment is obtainable from a doctor in England too (see *Appendix*).

At Carlsbad in Czechoslovakia, and at Trefriw Spa in North Wales, the natural spring water is curative because it is rich in iron. Dr. Vogel's remedy is whey-concentrate (MOLKOSAN), one teaspoonful mixed with the cereal. The biochemic tissue salt Nat. sulph. should be taken (5 pilules at bedtime).

DIARRHOEA

This is usually due to inflammation and irritation of the large bowel, producing too much lubricating mucus (possibly due to overdosing with laxatives for constipation). It can also be caused by viruses, bacteria, inability to digest carbohydrate foods properly (causing a too rapid passage of the food through the intestine, so that it is unable to absorb quickly enough the water contained in the food). Other causes are disturbance of the thyroid or adrenal glands, prolonged worry or anxiety, or colitis (see 'Colitis'). Malabsorption of fats due to malfunction of the pancreas can also cause a sort of diarrhoea.

Prolonged diarrhoea needs investigation in the form of bowel X-ray and/or sigmoidoscopy (examination of the intestine with a lighted tube). Most types of diarrhoea are short-lived if a dose of castor oil or a purging dose of Epsom salts is taken. This removes all irritants and poisons, leaving the bowel clean. The patient will be slightly constipated for a day or two, but this will soon right itself.

Diarrhoea is one of the ways in which Nature rids the body of noxious substances and poisons, and so it should never be suppressed with suppressive drugs. If it is very troublesome, a tablespoonful of brandy in a little soda-water may be taken at bedtime. Cups of gruel, made with powdered arrowroot and gum-arabic (acacia powder), should be sipped slowly at frequent intervals; it should be warm but not hot. Raw apple (grated or pulped), mixed with 1 teaspoonful of apple-pectin (made by British Drug Houses Ltd. and, like the arrowroot and the gum-arabic, obtainable from any good chemist), and, for a change, little drinks of malted milk (warm but not hot), can be taken instead of the arrowroot gruel.

Other helpful remedies include meadowsweet-herb tea, and drinks made with slippery-elm powder, to which is added 1 teaspoonful of bayberry powder, and 1 teaspoonful of cinnamon powder. At bedtime, a small pinch of powdered rhubarb-compound, plus a little honey, should be added to a drink of warm barley-water or arrowroot-gruel. Two Biochemic Ferrum. phos. pilules should be dissolved under the tongue 3 times a day.

If the diarrhoea is due to gastro-enteritis, the diet should include whey powder and Enpac tablets (see *Appendix*). A vitamin B.12 tablet should be taken 3 times a week.

For prolonged chronic diarrhoea, a few sips of tea, twice

a day, made with leaves of the Vinca-major plant (peri-winkle) are helpful.

Cow's milk is not recommended, either for adults or children; a better milk drink is Casilan made by Glaxo Laboratories, or Granogen (made by Granose Foods) using 1 heaped tablespoonful to ½ pint of tepid water. A little whey powder (which is mostly milk-sugar) can be added.

Infantile diarrhoea. A teaspoonful of raw tomato juice, at intervals of an hour or so, will remedy this. To 1 table-spoonful of yoghourt add 1 saltspoonful of carob-bean powder, and a little mashed-up banana, and give this every 4 hours. Carob-bean powder is made from the carob bean (see *Appendix*).

DIFFICULT MENSTRUATION (Dismenorrhoea)

This is sometimes due to a chill, and can be eased by sitting in hot water which reaches just up to the navel, at the same time sipping a cup of hot herb-tea made of pennyroyal and tansy herbs, sweetened with honey. The tea is made by pouring 1 pint of boiling water over 1 oz. each of the herbs, in a teapot. Stir well and allow it to infuse for 10 minutes. Then strain, warm up a cupful in a saucepan, add 2 drops of homoeopathic tincture of pulsatilla, sweeten with a little honey, and drink a little every 3 hours. Between periods, take motherwort-herb tea, made in exactly the same way. It should be taken (a wineglassful) 3 times a day, before meals. 'Calcium-plus' tablets should also be taken (3 a day).

Difficult menstruation can be due to an imbalance of sex hormones, and/or emotional disturbance, which *can* stop the periods entirely, if it is great enough.

DIGESTIVE DISORDERS

These are very fully explained and dealt with by Captain Frank Roberts, M.N.I.M.H., in his book *Encyclopaedia of*

Digestive Disorders (Thorsons Ltd.). The disorders include Colitis, Constipation, Duodenal Ulcer, Diverticulitis, etc.

DIPHTHERIA

Use Red-sage tea, both as a drink and as a gargle. The tea can be sweetened with honey, and a pinch of cinnamon added. To make the tea, pour 1 pint of boiling water over 1 oz. of red sage. Cover, and allow it to infuse for ½ hour; then strain, warm up, add the juice of half a lemon and a little honey, and sip slowly. Use it also as a gargle.

Pineapple juice is another good remedy; so, too, is neat lemon juice. The juice, allowed to trickle down the throat very slowly, will often prevent a membrane forming, or will cut it if it *has* formed.

A homoeopathic remedy is phytolacca, using 2–3 drops of the fresh tincture in a little warm water, as a gargle, every hour. The final mouthful each time can be swallowed.

A thick slice of toasted bread, soaked in very hot vinegar and wrapped in a large handkerchief, should be applied to the throat and kept in place by a stocking. The whole body should be rubbed over every day with vinegar; this supplies new electric tension to the nerve-endings, and draws stagnating blood to the surface, thereby improving circulation.

DISSEMINATED (MULTIPLE) SCLEROSIS

Owing to the fact that disseminated sclerosis is a disease of the fatty-protein covering of the nerves, and to the fact that it is unknown amongst the Eskimos, whose diet consists almost entirely of meat and fish (i.e. protein and fats), it is thought to be a disease due to a diet with a low content of protein and fats, and a high content of starches and sugars. This high-carbohydrate type of diet also causes low blood-pressure, and low blood-pressure very often accompanies sclerosis.

The diet of people with sclerosis should, therefore, have its protein and its fat-content stepped up, and its starch-sugar content reduced to a minimum. The protein should not be animal protein; cheese, eggs, milk and milk-products, yoghourt, nuts, seeds and soya-beans, lentils, etc., all provide first-class vegetable protein. Butter, cheese, milk, cream and yoghourt, provide animal fat; sunflower-seed oil, safflower-seed oil, corn-oil, soya-bean oil, nuts, and avocado pears, provide vegetable fat; this is essential because it provides a most important unsaturated fatty-acid, linoleic acid. Vitamin E (to counteract the wastage of oxygen produced by the digestion of the fats) should be included in the daily diet also.

Treatment should commence with a 2-day fast, during which time only raw vegetable-juices, fruit, and hot drinks (no solid food), should be taken. Whilst fasting, 1 heaped teaspoonful of Epsom salts in hot water should be taken first thing each morning, followed by a hot drink. This should purge the bowels of all waste-products and poisons.

After the fast (which should be repeated at intervals of 4–5 weeks) the diet should consist mainly of uncooked foods, i.e. raw vegetable juices, salads, and fruits (fresh and sun-dried), although cooked vegetables, especially *broad beans* (which contain a substance called Dopa L, invaluable in the treatment of this, and other nervous complaints) should be eaten. Salads and vegetables should be dressed with safflower-seed oil (rich in linoleic acid) and cider-vinegar (equal quantities). Bread, etc. made of wheat-flour should be avoided because of its high gluten content. Gluten-free bread and flour are obtainable. (See page 88.) Sugar should be replaced by honey entirely, table-salt by garlic powder, coffee by dandelion coffee, and alcoholic drinks by pure apple or grape juice (obtainable from most health-foods shops). Butter should be unsalted, and sunflower-seed oil margarine used instead of cooking-fats. Milk should be unpasteurized; if only pasteurized is obtainable, partly replace it with skim-milk, plantmilk or soya-bean milk. A large cupful of yoghourt (made with goat's milk and obtainable from most health-foods shops) should be eaten every day with dried fruit such as apricots, pears, peaches, or with baked apple. The dried fruit should be washed, then soaked in warm water overnight (or longer), but not cooked, and it will not need sweetening, having been sun-dried. A mashed-up ripe banana, covered with a few spoonfuls of soya-bean milk (Granogen), makes a complete meal.

Farmhouse or cottage cheese, also cheese-and-egg dishes, lentil savouries, and lentil soup (with onions and other vegetables), soya-beans, nuts and seeds (including sesame seeds, millet seeds, sunflower seeds and linseed) should take the place of meat and other flesh foods. The nuts and seeds must, of course, be ground up in a small nut-mill or coffee-mill.

A tablespoonful or two of barleygerm powder (Gestaal) to which has been added 1 teaspoonful of whey powder, 2–4 teaspoonfuls of powdered brewer's yeast (Yestamin), a salt-spoonful of vitamin C powder, and 2 vitamin E capsules, should be eaten with a little raw milk, plantmilk, or soya-bean milk, every day.

To make good any deficiency of vitamin B.12, and of 'trace-elements' in the diet, it is advisable to dissolve 3–4 kelp tablets and 3–4 alfalfa tablets in $\frac{1}{2}$ cupful of hot (vegetable) water, and to add this, together with 1 small tea-spoonful of unsalted 'Barmene' or Vecon, to the $\frac{1}{2}$ cupful of raw vegetable-juices. This should be taken shortly before the midday or evening meal.

Deep massage of the whole spine should be given daily, finally applying eucalyptus oil. Active and passive move-ments of the limbs should also be performed, following the massage. Deeper massage of the spine can be given by the operator by using his knee. For this, the patient sits on a low stool, with his/her back to the operator, arms supported on a low table, head resting on them.

To improve the circulation to, and through, the spinal cord, and to relieve congestion, 'Cupping' treatment should be given, or a Cantharides plaster applied to the whole spine. In *Some Unusual Methods of Healing* (Health Science Press) Mr. Leslie Korth, D.O., gives details of 'Cupping' therapy; also of Pyonex treatment, which is often beneficial.

Biochemic Kali. phos. (potassium phosphate) should be taken; also biochemic Silica. The dose is 5 pilules of silica 6x. in the forenoon, and 5 pilules of Kali. phos. at bedtime. The pilules must be allowed to dissolve slowly under the tongue. Homoeopathic Hypericum 30. (5 pilules twice daily) should also be taken.

Worry, stress, noise, and strain *must* be avoided, and as much rest taken as possible. Given rest, quiet, freedom from worry and stress, and the right foods, together with the other forms of treatment suggested, or Dr. Samuel's short-wave treatment (see *Appendix*), the condition can be prevented from getting any worse, and indeed is nearly sure to improve.

DIVERTICULITIS

This is an inflammation of diverticula (pockets or bulges in the intestinal wall where the wall is muscularly weak), causing pain and discomfort on the left side of the abdomen, and accompanied usually by constipation (sometimes by diarrhoea), occasionally by bleeding from the bowel, and sometimes (though rarely) by complete stoppage of the bowels.

If the condition persists and becomes chronic, the lower bowel should be X-rayed and investigated by sigmoidoscopy (inspection with a lighted tube).

People with diverticulitis should avoid rough foods; on the other hand, they need 'bulk' (everyone does). This is best provided by bran. A finely-milled bran is made by Allinsons, the flour millers. Breakfast should consist of finely-milled bran, prunes soaked overnight in water containing molasses, mashed-up banana, honey, and yoghourt. Surgical removal of the affected part of the intestine is resorted to only for very severe or complicated cases.

DIZZINESS (Vertigo)

This can be due to such a variety of causes that it is well-nigh impossible to suggest remedies, because always treatment depends upon the underlying cause. This can be liver derangement, high (or low) blood-pressure, over-strain, or worry, under-nourishment, malnutrition, low blood-sugar, anaemia and general weakness, a sudden rush of blood to the head, and a thousand and one other things. Try taking little drinks of cider-vinegar and water ($\frac{1}{2}$ teaspoonful in $\frac{1}{2}$ cupful of water) at bedtime, every night, and again next morning. After a few days, make the dose 1 teaspoonful. If this does not cure the giddiness, try taking biochemic Kali. phos. (3 pilules at bedtime) and, if anaemic, Ferrum phos. (3 pilules after meals). Drink rutin-herb tea, and attend to your bowel movements (see 'Constipation'). Exercise in the fresh air every day, eat natural, mostly raw, foods, and above all do not worry. Worry upsets the glands, and glandular imbalance can cause dizziness. Get your blood-pressure taken, and your blood tested for anaemia.

DROPSY

This is a typical 'impurities' disease, caused by an accumulation of waste products in the blood – an accumulation so great that the kidneys and liver become overloaded and unable to perform their purifying tasks properly. The stagnation of unhealthy fluids in the tissues can, also, be aggravated and increased by the heart muscle being too weak to pump the blood with sufficient force through the veins and arteries to carry the necessary oxygen and nourishment to the cells of the vital organs. The result of such weak pumping action is stagnation of the body-fluids and poisoning of the whole system. Such a condition can be cured by detoxication of the body by means of a semi-fasting cleansing diet, bowel wash-outs, and heart stimulating remedies.

When there is heart weakness, a complete fast should not be undertaken; it involves the risk of further weakening, but a semi-fast may be safely undertaken, and, together with nightly enemas to cleanse the bowels, and doses of a homoeopathic heart-remedy, tincture of Crataegus, will rapidly detoxicate the whole body.

The semi-fast means a daily diet on the following lines: An early-morning fresh lemon drink, or apple-juice, or a wineglassful of pure grape-juice. No solid food should be taken before midday. Lunch should consist of 1–2 potatoes cooked in their skins, runner-beans as often as possible, a raw mixed salad (the salad dressed with lemon-juice and olive oil); 1 round of wholewheat bread or toast, with a very thin scraping of butter on it; a little cottage cheese or lactic-acid cream cheese (no other sort), followed by egg-custard or milk jelly made with 'Gelozone'. The water in which the beans have been cooked should be mixed with raw carrot juice, and drunk before the meal. The evening meal should be a repetition of this lunch meal. About half an hour after the evening meal, a warm-water 1-pint enema should be given, and during the first week of treatment, a similar small enema should be given in the morning as well.

Sometimes, in more advanced cases of dropsy, it becomes necessary to draw off some of the unhealthy fluid that has collected in the tissues, and after this has been done great relief is experienced, but this is short-lived and the 'puncture' has to be repeated again and again, unless, at the same time, the diet is reformed. Orthodox medical treatment of dropsy – i.e. the drawing off of fluid – is good, as far as it goes, but it does not go far enough; it should include instructions about what, and what not, to eat and drink. The wrong foods hamper the healing powers of the body, and cause the fluid to re-form. For instance, no salt or salted foods should be eaten, and no soporifics or sleeping-drugs taken, as these inhibit the excretion of urine and thus favour water-retention. Excess sodium chloride (salt) causes water-retention; Dr. Gilbert's biochemic remedy, 'Chlorena', removes it.

The herbal remedy is a herb-tea made of the following herbs:

Equisetum (horsetail)	$\frac{1}{2}$ oz.
Rosemary	$\frac{1}{2}$ oz.
Broom tops	$\frac{1}{2}$ oz.
Buchu leaves	$\frac{1}{2}$ oz.
Dandelion root	$\frac{1}{2}$ oz.
Squill	$\frac{1}{2}$ oz.
Juniper berries	$\frac{1}{2}$ oz.

Stew the herbs gently in 2 pints of water for about 45 minutes. Strain; add the juice of a lemon and a little honey, and take a small drink of the mixture every 2 hours. Drinks of honey-sweetened water to which a pinch of cream of tartar has been added, should also be taken.

Homoeopathic Phaseolus 12 (derived from runner-beans) should be taken; the dose is 5 pilules mid-morning. If there is heart-weakness, fluid extract of convallaria (lily-of-the-valley) is helpful; the dose is 10 drops in a little water, before meals. Vitamin E capsules (1 with meals) are essential (see *Building a Healthy Heart*, by Eric Powell, N.D., Health Science Press).

DUODENAL ULCER

An ulcer is Nature's way of repairing the damage done by an over-abundance of hydrochloric acid in the stomach, which burns the delicate lining of the stomach. This acid would do less damage if natural unrefined foods were eaten, because the high-protein content of these foods acts as a buffer between the strong acid and the delicate lining. Refined foods have been stripped of their protein content, so over-abundant stomach-acids attack the stomach itself.

Treatment for the first 2–3 days. Rest in bed, taking only Biobalm, Casilan, orange juice in milk, comfrey-herb tea, Malvern spring-water, raw carrot-juice, cabbage-juice, potato-juice, celery-juice, and potato water. About 1 table-spoonful of the vegetable-juices should be taken (with 1

116

tablespoonful of water), every 2 hours, and 1 tablespoonful of raw potato juice last thing at night.

Potato water is made as follows: Scrub and cut up, but do not peel, about 1 lb. of potatoes. Plunge them into about 1½ pints of unsalted boiling water; boil them gently for about ½ hour, then strain, allow to cool, and drink a little of the water at frequent intervals. It should be made fresh every day.

A 1-pint warm-water enema should be given every day, to clear the lower bowel of all effete matter. Later, when more solid food is being eaten, the enema should be used less frequently and should gradually become unnecessary. If the bowel is ulcerated, a tablespoonful of Kaolin is added to the enema water, and 1 teaspoonful of linseed oil should be taken once a day, in an orange-milk drink.

Treatment for the next 10 days. The diet should now include the following: Drinks of Biobalm food-beverage, carrot juice, cabbage juice, potato water, cooked potato and cooked carrots mashed up with a trickle of vegetable oil; ripe banana mashed up with a little milk and 1 spoonful of whey powder, rusks or Ryvita biscuits. A little, and often, is best.

Treatment after 2 weeks. The following foods may be added to the diet: grated raw apple; grated raw carrot; cooked spinach; malted milk, soya-bean milk, plantmilk, and raw egg-yolk.

The Biobalm food-beverage, which contains slippery-elm and malt, and is a medicine as well as a food, can now be made with more milk than water and a little milk-sugar (lactose) added. A little milk-sugar (lactose) may also be added to the other drinks. Whey powder is rich in lactose and can be obtained from the Biochemic Centre (see *Appendix*). It is *not* the same thing as glucose.

After a few more days, the following may be added to the diet: St. Ivel or cottage cheese, a little unsalted butter, and a slice or two of home-made bread (toasted), baked potato in its skin, yolk of egg (discard the white), baked egg-yolk custard (without added sugar), ripe tomato, tender lettuce, sweet ripe grapes, baked apple stuffed with dates. If any one of these additions causes discomfort and a return of the pain, it should be omitted. It is best to 'go slow' at first, trying fresh additions one at a time, and discarding any new one that causes the slightest discomfort.

Flesh foods are best omitted permanently from the diet. Fried and fatty foods should be avoided; also all forms of sugar except honey, milk-sugar (whey), sun-dried fruit (such as dates, raisins, etc.) which contains natural fruit-sugar (fructose), sweet raw apple, and sweet ripe grapes. Ripe bananas may be eaten, but not the usual green-cum-yellow variety seen in greengrocer's shops; these are picked before they are ripe and might be indigestible. Tree-ripened bananas (dried and packeted) are obtainable from many of the health-foods shops. Other things to avoid are white flour and white-flour products (i.e. white bread, cakes, biscuits, etc.), refined white cereals (white rice, white barley, etc.), all processed foods, all hot or highly-spiced foods, all condiments including pepper, salt, and mustard (use kelp powder, garlic powder, and celery powder instead), strong tea, coffee, alcohol, and smoking. Dandelion coffee should replace ordinary coffee, and comfrey-herb tea or yarrow-herb tea mixed with English herb tea (which contains meadowsweet) should replace ordinary tea.

To heal completely, the ulcer may take anything from 1 month to 18 months, so great patience and perseverance is needed; also self-discipline. And, of course, there may be times when the symptoms return. But do not despair; simply go back to raw juices and Biobalm for a few days, and suck vegetable-charcoal tablets if the pain is bad. In time, the ulcer *will* heal. When it does, the diet must then be built up to include more vegetable-protein, more vitamin- and mineral-rich foods such as salads, raw vegetables, and fresh fruit.

Extensive information re duodenal ulcer and its curative treatment can be found in *The Herbal Cure of Duodenal Ulcers* by Captain Frank Roberts, M.C., M.N.I.M.H. The book, also tablets made to his own special formula, are available from him direct. (His address is The Herbal Dispensaries, Hanham, Near Bristol.)

The herbal formula is as follows:

Tincture of Echinacea	3½ oz.
Tincture of Phytolacca	3½ oz.
Fluid extract of Marshmallow root	3½ oz.
Fluid extract of Golden Seal root	3½ oz.
Fluid extract of Cranesbill root	3½ oz.

The above remedy is available from Captain Roberts in tablet or liquid form. It should be taken as directed on the bottle.

DYSENTERY

This is an exaggerated form of diarrhoea (sometimes brought on by getting chilled after perspiring heavily), in which the toxic state of the bowels provides a breeding-ground for certain germs. A lack of iron in the walls of the blood vessels causes haemorrhage and inflammation, so that blood and mucus come away in the stools. It is characterized by straining and cramp-like pains in the abdomen and bowels.

There will be no desire for solid food, but the sufferer should take a little calves' foot jelly (lemon-flavoured), and 'Biobalm' food-beverage, to which a pinch of flowers-of-sulphur and a teaspoonful of acacia powder (gum-arabic) has been added, at 4-hourly intervals, with drinks of herbal tea in between. The herbs used for the tea should be dried nettles, shepherd's purse, and cranesbill, using 1 oz. of each to 2 pints of boiling water. Allow the tea to stand for 30 minutes; then strain, add a teaspoonful of bayberry-herb powder, re-heat, and drink a cupful. Milk and honey may be

119

added. Other drinks should include raw carrot-juice, raw apple-juice, and raw lemon-juice in honeyed water. Raw apples, pears, bilberries, blackberries, strawberries (when in season) may be eaten, as they are all strongly astringent.

Oil of garlic capsules (1 before each 4-hourly feed) should be taken. Biochemic mag. phos. 6x. can be taken for the pain, every half-hour if necessary.

A homoeopathic remedy for dysentery is Ipececuanha 30. (5 pilules at bedtime), but a homoeopathic doctor should prescribe.

The whole body should be frictioned all over with luke-warm vinegar water, at least once a day.

Earache

Apply hot cloths, or rest the affected side of the head on a rubber hot water bottle. A few drops of warmed honey or almond oil, dropped into the ear with a fountain-pen filler or glass dropper, will give speedy relief. A homoeopathic remedy is Lachesis 30, but a homoeopathic doctor should be consulted. (See also 'Catarrh'.)

Eczema

Remedies to purify the blood are needed. Take homoeopathic tincture of echinacea 2x. (10–15 drops in a spoonful of water 3 times daily); also a herbal tea made with equal parts of sarsaparilla root, yellow-dock root, burdock root, and poke-root (1 tablespoonful 3 times daily after meals).

A cleansing diet should be eaten – a diet that includes plenty of green leafy vegetables and salads, especially water-cress, and raw vegetable juices, especially carrots, cucumber and nettles. When these are out of season, they can be obtained in dehydrated powdered form (see Remedial Products in the *Appendix*). Dress salads with vegetable oil (sunflower-seed or soya-bean).

Watercress juice, applied externally to the patches of eczema, will relieve irritation and may even cure the trouble.

When fresh watercress is not available, dried powdered watercress may be used (moistened). Rumex ointment is also helpful.

Eczema caused by bacteria. Salt and salted foods should be eliminated; a little bicarbonate of potash can take the place of table-salt. Consumption of bread should be drastically reduced; rye bread is preferable to wheat-bread. A preparation containing usnic acid (made from beard-lichen) should be applied.

Weeping eczema. For this, take the herbal tea recommended for Dropsy.

EMPHYSEMA

See 'Bronchitis', also 'Catarrh'.

ENTERITIS

Nettle tea is a good remedy (see 'Dysentery'). Use dried skim-milk powder, and 'Granogen' soya-milk powder instead of cow's milk. Use honey or whey powder instead of ordinary sugar. (See 'Bowel Troubles'.)

EPILEPSY

The herbal remedy is mistletoe tea, using 2 oz. of the herb to $\frac{1}{2}$ pint of boiling water. The biochemic remedy is Kali. phos. 6x. A homoeopathic remedy is Sambuccus niger 3x. (elder-flower), although in some cases Peony officinalis 3x. is more effective. To go to Carlsbad and drink the waters would be very beneficial.

EYE TROUBLES

People with weak eyesight, or sore and inflamed eyes, should use an eye-lotion made as follows: To 2 tablespoonfuls of rose-water and 1 tablespoonful of plain (boiled) water, add 5 drops of tincture of euphrasia. It can be bought ready-made from some health-foods shops under the name of 'eyebright' lotion.

For grit in the eye (or any other foreign body), drop 1 drop of castor oil into the eye with a fountain-pen filler.

For scaly eyelids, take a teaspoonful (or more) of vegetable oil every day on salads or vegetables.

For follicles on the eyelid, used fireweed ointment.

For cataract, take homoeopathic Calcarea Iodide 6.

FEVERISHNESS

A fevered state is caused by a fermenting disintegration of the albuminous substances in the blood, and can be reduced by taking frequent sips of $\frac{1}{2}$ pint of warm water, to which a teaspoonful of cider-vinegar has been added; also by taking frequent sips of a quart of cold boiled water to which $\frac{1}{8}$ oz. of Glaubers salts and $\frac{1}{8}$ oz. of common salt has been added (a quart is sufficient for 2 days). Biochemic Ferrum. phos. should be taken (3 pilules every 4 hours) alternating with Kali. mur. pilules. The body should be sponged all over once or twice a day with vinegar and water.

As the fever abates, sips of warm milk, in which a pinch of flowers of sulphur is dissolved, may be taken; also almond-milk made of a mixture of ground sweet almonds (4 oz.), gum-arabic ($\frac{1}{2}$ oz.), a little honey, and $\frac{1}{2}$ pint of warm water. Hot lemonade, with added honey and gum-arabic, may be taken from the start; also a herb-tea made of yarrow and boneset, and citrus fruit-juices. It is essential to rest in bed until the fever goes.

FLATULENCE

This may be due to insufficient hydrochloric acid in the stomach, resulting from a lack of folic acid (one of the B vitamins manufactured in the intestines); anaemia can cause this; the remedy is to eat foods rich in B vitamins, especially brewer's yeast, wheatgerm, and green leafy vegetables. If this does not help, one capsule of glutamic-acid hydrochloride should be taken after each meal. This will supply the missing hydrochloric acid, though not the missing folic acid; brewer's yeast should therefore be part of the daily diet. Garlic is a good digestive; it can be eaten in dried powder form, sprinkled on to vegetables and into raw vegetable-juices, or taken in homoeopathic pilule form (its homoeopathic name is Allium sativum).

Vegetable-charcoal tablets are also helpful; they absorb stomach gases resulting from fermentation of foods in the stomach – usually incompatible foods (see 'Compatible and Incompatible Foods'). So, too, is a pinch of ground-up nutmeg in hot water, before meals.

Suspected lack of hydrochloric acid in the stomach can nowadays be tested by measurement of an enzyme in the urine. This should certainly be made, especially in cases of anaemia where food is obviously not being properly assimilated and the sufferer is therefore thin and under-nourished, as well as suffering from indigestion and flatulence.

Bowel flatulence can be relieved by taking whey powder, or, better still, Florus powder (see *Appendix*).

The remedy for chronic flatulence is Nux. mosch (nutmeg). The dose is 5 pilules before meals, for several weeks.

GALLSTONES

The main causes are faulty feeding, over-eating (with consequent obesity), lack of physical exercise, and a consequent lack of bile secretion by the liver, which means that there is insufficient bile to deal with the over-abundance of food that has been eaten (especially of animal fats and animal-proteins). Over-eating or faulty feeding (or both) causes an imbalance of cholesterol and bile salts in the gallbladder, and this leads to the formation of gallstones, which are made almost entirely of cholesterol.

An inadequate secretion of bile by the liver, due usually to lack of physical exercise, means that insufficient bile is poured (via the gall-bladder where it is stored) into the intestines, for emulsifying the large globules of fat, and for removing the layers of fat that cover the protein and carbohydrate foods eaten. The amount of bile becomes doubly insufficient if the amount of food eaten has been more than is required by the body.

The insufficiency of bile means that all food eaten in excess of normal bodily requirements remains undigested in the intestines, because the digestive enzymes in the intestines cannot penetrate the layers of fat covering the food, nor can they themselves break down the fatty layers nor the large fat globules. This undigested food encourages the growth of putrefactive bacteria which produce putrefactive gas, malodorous flatulence, bowel-toxaemia, indigestion, and great discomfort. A lack of normal bile in the intestines will also cause constipation, headache, and a feeling of general malaise, and, of course, the stones that may form in the gallbladder will cause pain and will block the free flow of bile, both to and from the gall-bladder.

Orthodox operative treatment removes the stones (the cause of bile-blockage) – sometimes the whole gall-bladder is removed – but it does not remove the *cause* of the trouble, i.e. the over-eating, the lack of exercise, etc., and, if these are not dealt with, they will set up trouble elsewhere in the body, possibly of a more serious nature.

Nature-cure treatment consists of fasting for two or three days on fresh fruit-juices (excluding orange); pear wine (Perry) and apple-juice, also grapefruit juice (in hot water), are particularly beneficial. So long as there is pain, no solid food should be eaten, and, even when it has gone, the diet should consist of juices only, for a further 2–3 days. After that, malted milk may be taken every 3–4 hours; also fresh fruit.

During this first week of treatment, a warm water enema, given daily, helps to relieve pain and cleanses the bowels.

Hot linseed-meal or bran poultices should be applied to the painful area frequently. A teaspoonful of best (cold-pressed) olive oil should be well shaken in a jar, together with the juice of half a lemon, and taken twice a day. The shaking-up emulsifies the oil and makes it tasteless and easily digested.

When a solid-food diet is resumed, it should exclude flesh foods, cut down animal fats and starch-and-sugar foods, and consist mainly of vegetables, salads (especially radishes), fresh (and dried) fruits, nuts and seeds, cottage cheese, wholewheat bread, etc. Leeks, and the water in which they are cooked, are very beneficial. So, too, are dandelion coffee and parsley-piert herb tea. Things should be sweetened with honey, not sugar. A good homoeopathic remedy is Choleterin 30 (5 pills night and morning). Lecithin tablets should be taken 3 times a day (one with each meal), to emulsify the cholesterol.

GOUT

This is sometimes due to over-indulgence in alcoholic liquors, but more often it is due to eating too much meat, too much starch-and-sugar foods, and too little fresh fruit and vegetables. In other words, to eating too much cooked dead food, and not enough raw live food.

If the sufferer is overweight, he should fast for a day or two on fresh fruit and vegetable-juices, and take drinks every 2 or 3 hours of herbal teas such as goutwort-herb tea, parsley tea, nettle tea, alpine-herb tea, and hot lemonade (unsweetened), the idea being to flush the kidneys thoroughly. Dry cider or apple-juice is also helpful.

If underweight, the drinks may be supplemented by an apple or two, but no other food should be eaten for 24–48 hours. During this period, a herbal laxative such as Innerfresh should be taken at bedtime, and a saltspoonful dose of Glaubers salts next morning, followed by a hot bath in which 1 lb. of common Epsom salts is dissolved. This, followed by skin-friction with a rough towel, will help elimination of toxins through the skin. Massage, with deep frictions to the lumbar region of the back, should follow, as it is thought that gout originates in the lumbar region. The painful joint can be poulticed with warmed honey spread on a pad of lint that has been wrung out in hot nettle tea or goutwort-herb tea.

The short fast (on liquids only) should be followed for a few days by a diet of baked potato, toast, and barley-water, with apples, grapes, and vegetable juices taken between meals. A little unsalted butter may be eaten with the toast, and the barley-water may be sweetened with honey. Sugar should be entirely eliminated from the diet; also table-salt. A little Bio-salt may be taken with salads etc., which should include radishes, watercress, dandelion, tomato, and carrots. Potato-water and nettle tea are valuable drinks. (For recipe, see page 199.) When in season, cherries should be eaten daily.

To prevent further attacks, take a pinch of Glaubers salts in your early-morning tea every day. Signs of a recurring attack can often be successfully staved off by fasting for a day or two on cherries and apples only.

There are several good homoeopathic remedies. They are:

Urtica Urens 3x. (stinging nettle), which aids elimination of uric acid and eases skin irritation.

Ledum 3x. (wild rosemary), which eases sore and tender feet.

Phaseolus 12x. (runner-beans), which helps elimination of acids through its cleansing action on the kidneys and bladder.

The biochemic remedy is Nat. sulph. (Glaubers salts) taken in alternation with Ferrum. phos. Take ¼ teaspoonful of the salts in hot water (or tea) on rising, and 5 pilules of Ferrum. phos. at bedtime. These, and the homoeopathic pilules, should be allowed to dissolve slowly under the tongue, not swallowed whole. Allopurinol is the orthodox medical remedy.

GOITRE

Simple goitre is an enlargement of the thyroid gland, caused by a lack of iodine in the diet. Without iodine, the gland cannot produce its Thyroxine hormone, the hormone that controls the rate at which the body burns up its food – the rate at which it 'ticks over', so to speak. In its effort to produce sufficient Thyroxine, in the absence of sufficient iodine, it enlarges, and may become very large and unsightly and have to be removed surgically. The lack of iodine can be remedied by taking 1 drop of Lugol's solution in a little water or vegetable-juices, every other day, before a meal. Iodine is found in all sea-foods and in seaweed (kelp), in watercress, onions, and all green vegetables. Green vegetables (especially sprouts) also contain calcium, a mineral that goitre people often lack. Other foods rich in calcium are yoghourt, goat's milk, almonds, and cheese.

Brewer's yeast should be taken for its content of B vitamins.

A homoeopathic remedy is Equisetum 30 (5 pilules night and morning).

The biochemic remedy Calcium phos. 12x. will remedy calcium shortage.

Toxic goitre (*Graves' disease*) is over-activity of the thyroid gland. There may be very little, if any, swelling. The symptoms are an over-rapid burning up of the body's fuel, so that, due to lack of nourishment, the body loses weight; the heart becomes over-active and its beat irregular; the patient becomes restless and irritable.

The over-activity of the gland is due to an excess of the normal thyroid-stimulating hormone produced by the pituitary gland, or to an *abnormal* hormone coming from the hypothalmus gland. If due to the latter, the eyes of the patient protrude, and the complaint is known as *Exophthalmic goitre*. In both cases, iodine may help for a time, but usually toxic goitre and exophthalmic goitre have to be treated surgically (removal of part of the gland). But before surgery, the over-production of Thyroxine, which is causing an over-active heart must be damped down; otherwise the operation might be dangerous. Rest, and doses of iodine, or of a drug such as Thiourea, should be given for a few weeks, as a preparation for operation. An alternative to surgery is treatment of the pituitary gland by short-wave, as given by Dr. Jules Samuels of Amsterdam (see *Appendix*). Sometimes the iodine-and-drug treatment cures without an operation. So does the short-wave treatment.

GROWTHS

The late Dr. Forbes-Ross, author of *Cancer, its Genesis and Treatment*, advised people who fear that they may develop a growth to take a pinch of bicarbonate of potash every day, in ½ glassful of hot water, on rising, and to use black molasses (rich in potassium), instead of sugar. The late Dr. Kirstin Nolfi, author of *The Raw Food Treatment of Cancer and Other Diseases*, advocated fasting on vegetable-juices only, for several weeks, followed by many weeks (or months) of an entirely raw-foods diet. Her advice is based upon the fact that only raw foods contain vitally-important vitamins and enzymes – that heat-treatment (cooking) destroys vitamins (or, at any rate, alters them), and that growths occur when the body is deficient in vitamins and enzymes. Air-pollution, food-processing, and food-refining also destroy vitamins and enzymes; that is why it is so important to breathe pure fresh air at all times, and to eat only fresh natural foods rather than packaged, processed, preserved, or frozen ones.

External tumours, also polypus in the nose, should be treated by application of bloodroot-herb (powdered).

HAEMORRHOIDS (Piles)

This is an ailment that is associated with the taking of purgatives for constipation, and a toxic state of the blood due to faulty feeding. It can be cured by attention to diet; neither operation nor injection of the veins is necessary or advisable.

A diet on the following lines is suggested:

On rising, the juice of half a lemon in hot water (with molasses to sweeten).

Breakfast, soak some ground-up grains of oats (groats) in a little boiling water for 15 minutes; add wheatgerm, All-bran, a few prunes, some prune-juice containing a teaspoonful of molasses, a teaspoonful of powdered Agar-agar, and a little plantmilk. (The prunes should be soaked overnight in warm water, to which a teaspoonful of molasses has been added; they will not need cooking.) A cup of dandelion coffee may follow. Plums, when in season, can replace prunes.

Midday meal, a salad consisting of lettuce, watercress, tomato, dandelion leaves, parsley, etc., preceded by a wine-glassful of raw carrot juice (or mixed vegetable juices), the salad to be dressed with soya-bean oil and cider-vinegar. A potato cooked in its skin, wholewheat bread or toast, a little butter and some cottage cheese, followed by sun-dried fruit (apricots, peaches, pears, figs, dates, etc.) or mashed-up *ripe* banana with goat's-milk yoghourt.

Evening meal, a cereal consisting of a mixture of ground-up nuts and seeds (sunflower seeds, linseed, millet, sesame seed, almonds, cashew nuts, brazil nuts, etc., wheatgerm, a teaspoonful of wheatgerm oil, moistened with a little soya-bean milk (reconstituted), followed by a serving of conservatively-cooked vegetables (green vegetables, carrots, onions, and leeks are all especially valuable) together with poached or scrambled egg, wholewheat bread or toast. (Grated cheese or nut-rissole can replace the egg sometimes.) The water in which the vegetables have been cooked contains valuable minerals; it should be conserved, flavoured with a little 'Vecon', and taken with raw vegetable-juices half an hour before a meal. Sweets can consist of baked custard and a mashed-up *ripe* banana, or some dates, or sultanas and raisins.

Daily exercise in the fresh air is *very* important; brisk walking is the best exercise, but swimming is also very good; both forms of exercise deepen the breathing and strengthen the abdominal muscles, which are usually weak and flabby. In addition, the following abdominal exercises should be done every day, for about 5 minutes:

1. Lying flat on the floor, with a small pillow under the head, relax and de-tense every muscle in the body, breathing deeply and quietly.
2. Lying flat on the floor, with the toes tucked under the wardrobe or other heavy object (to anchor them) raise the upper part of the body to sitting position, then let it fall back slowly to the floor. Repeat several times.
3. Lying flat, raise both legs to a vertical position, keeping the knees unbent; then lower the legs to the floor, slowly and steadily, without letting the head rise up off the floor. (This is more difficult than it sounds.) Repeat several times.
4. Standing, grasp the back of a chair, bend the knees, expelling the breath at the same time. Resume the upright position as you breathe in. Repeat 3–4 times.

Mental and emotional tension, especially worry, causes muscular tension. This causes a loss of nervous energy, which leads to constipation – one of the chief causes of piles. So try not to be a worrier; your piles will get better more quickly if you do not worry about them. Deep breathing done gently – in through the nose, out through the mouth on a long-drawn sigh – helps muscular relaxation.

Sitting down for long periods at a time is as detrimental

as long standing. Rest in the 'body-slant' position (feet up and supported on a surface higher than your heart, e.g. the mantelshelf) whenever you get the opportunity, if only for a few minutes. Also, push a bolster underneath the foot of the mattress, so that, when in bed, your feet and lower legs are slightly raised.

Neither surgical cutting of the veins, nor injecting them, deals with the underlying cause of the condition. If this is not dealt with by natural methods such as those briefly outlined above, the normal veins which remain, after the affected veins have been removed or injected, will in time become varicosed too, and there will then be a recurrence of the trouble. The treatment of the affected veins with electricity (negative galvanism) is preferable to cutting or injecting them.

Protruding piles should be gently pushed back into the rectum, using a clean forefinger soaped with pure Castile soap, whilst sitting in the bath. After the bath, sit on the edge of the bath (backwards) and bathe the area with hot water, finishing with cold water; then anoint the piles with fresh lemon-juice. At night, bathe again, anoint them with green pilewort or garlic ointment, and take a dose of the fluid-extract of pilewort (1 teaspoonful in a little hot water). Every morning and evening a dose of the following herbal mixture should be taken:

Fluid Extract of Collinsonia	4 oz.
Syrup (or Elixir) of Podophyllum	2 oz.
Extract of Witch-hazel	4 oz.

The biochemic remedy is Calc. fluor. 6x. before meals and Ferrum phos. 6x. after meals (3 pilules of each).

Itching piles can be eased by taking homoeopathic sulphur 6x. (2 pilules between meals).

The sufferer should read *Encyclopaedia of Digestive Disturbances* by Frank Roberts, M.C., M.N.I.M.H., in which the treatment of haemorrhoids (both internal and external) is dealt with very fully.

HAIR (Falling Out or Thinning)

The scalp should be massaged nightly with a mixture of Jaborandi and bay-rum. Once a week, massage the scalp with warmed oil of rosemary. Shampoo next day with warm rain-water and slippery-elm soap. To take biochemic Silica 6x. is sometimes helpful (2 pilules after meals). Diet is all-important, and hats should be discarded. (See 'Baldness'.)

HAY-FEVER

About 2 months before your annual attack usually comes on, start eating honeycomb every day. This will lessen the severity of the attack, if it does not entirely avert it. If and when the attack does start, the symptoms will be less severe if you fast for a day or two on fruit only, resting as much as possible to conserve energy, and take homoeopathic Allium cepa 30 (onion) or Sabadilla 30. The dose is 3 pilules every $\frac{1}{2}$ hour, till relieved. Camomile flowers (dried, set alight on a shovel, will smoulder and give off a smoke which, if inhaled, will soothe and relieve the nasal mucous membranes. Use powdered Bayberry bark as snuff. It will cause sneezing at first, but will harden the mucous membrane.

Hay-fever can be due to a diet deficient in vitamins and minerals, especially vitamin A and calcium, so take 'Calcium-Plus' tablets, and Pro-vitamin A capsules, and eat green salads, dressed with sunflower-seed oil and cider-vinegar, together with farmhouse cheese, an egg, whole-wheat bread, and unsalted butter. Yoghourt (made of goat's milk) is rich in calcium, and should be eaten with sun-dried apricots (soaked overnight but not cooked). Eat also whey powder, sprinkled over wheatgerm cereal and moistened with plantmilk. Flesh foods should be omitted, or drastically reduced. Cut down milk, also starch and sugar foods and eat more vegetables, raw vegetable-juices, salads, and fruit. Honey should take the place of sugar entirely, and table-salt should be replaced by garlic powder, onion powder, and celery powder. Kelp tablets (3–4 daily) should be ground up and added to raw vegetable juices. No aluminium cooking-vessels should be used.

A herbal remedy for hay-fever is tea made with Euphrasia herb, commonly called 'Eyebright'. (See *Nature-cure for Hay-fever and Asthma*, by Russell Sneddon (Gateway Book Co.).

Biochemic remedies are Ferrum. phos. 6x. (2 pilules before meals), Nat. mur. 6x. (2 pilules after meals), Kali. phos. 6x. at bedtime, and Nat. sulph. 6x. (or a pinch of Glaubers salts) on rising.

HEADACHE

There are so many disorders of which headache is a symptom that, without a thorough investigation, only the symptoms can be treated. A good general remedy, both for congestive and nervous headache, is the herb Melilotus; fresh tincture of Melilotus is obtainable from a homoeopathic chemist; the dose is 5 drops in 1 tablespoonful of water, every 15 minutes, till relieved. It can also be taken for sick headache (with or without indigestion and flatulence), and for throbbing headache. For neuralgic headache, take homoeopathic Gelsemium 30, or Cyclamen, or Aconitum 30. Apply spirits of camphor or a cold compress of vinegar on a folded handkerchief to the back of the neck and to the forehead. For migraine headache, take Cyclamen Opiz. (See *Appendix*.) A hot footbath and hot cloths applied to the anus will give relief.

Brewer's yeast should be included in the daily diet, and 1 vitamin B.12 tablet should be taken every other day. Biral is a good daytime sedative. (See *Appendix*.)

HEART TROUBLES

Most heart conditions, whether they are organic or purely functional, nearly always arise as secondary effects. Treatment, therefore, will vary according to the primary causation. For instance, a poor quality and wrongly-balanced diet may cause a liver or gall-bladder condition. In time, this condition may start to operate as a secondary cause, giving rise to subsequent heart disturbance, which would then be a secondary effect. In this case, to treat just the heart condition could never lead to permanent improvement, and a change-over to wholesome and balanced feeding would, therefore, be a basic necessity in order to normalize the faulty liver condition (the real primary cause). If *the liver* is suspect, it would be wise to omit eggs, oranges, chocolate, cream, and flesh foods, from the diet. (See 'Liver troubles'.)

If the trouble is of *kidney* origin, flesh foods should be replaced by vegetable-protein foods such as nuts, beans (especially soya-beans), lentils, cheese and eggs, wheatgerm, and brewer's yeast. Kelp (powdered seaweed) is rich in iodine and should replace salt entirely.

If the *blood-pressure* is high, animal fats (butter, milk and cream) and hydrogenated fats (lard, margarine, etc.) should be wholly replaced by nut-butter, nut-creams, corn-oil margarine, plantmilk, soya-bean milk, and yoghourt.

If chronic *bronchial or lung conditions* are involved, starches, sugars and cow's milk should be drastically reduced, because these foods tend to form catarrh.

If *indigestion* and flatulence is present, omit all indigestible things such as fried foods, twice-cooked foods, etc. and cut down on butter, cream, and other animal fats. Replace with vegetable fats.

Thyroid diysfunction may also be responsible for heart troubles. A remedy for this is 1 drop of medicinal iodine in a little milk, twice a week. It is often the result of pituitary gland disfunction, and this can be treated by Dr. Samuel's short-wave therapy. (See *Appendix*.)

The suppressive drugs used by the orthodox medical profession in the treatment of fevers (especially salicylates used in rheumatic ailments) are largely responsible for damage caused to the heart. Such ailments, if treated by Nature-cure methods, do not leave harmful after-effects on the heart (or any other organ).

Aspirin is another of the harmful drugs used to suppress feverish conditions and pain. This, and all other drugs, should be avoided by heart sufferers.

Certain drugs are known to have a definite effect upon the heart's action. Two of these – digitalis and strychnine – are prescribed by the medical profession, the first one for retarding the heart's action, the second for increasing it. But these drugs do not touch the cause of the trouble; at best they are purely palliative, and in the long run they do more harm than good.

In orthodox medical circles, the diet-factor is usually ignored, and heart conditions are considered incurable, whereas Nature-cure can help heart sufferers, no matter what the cause of the trouble, nor what the extent of the damage done by drugs or by wrong feeding may be. Of course, where the heart structures or valves are seriously damaged, a cure is impossible, though even here much can be done to alleviate, and to improve the condition. But, where the damage is only slight, or where it is due to functional rather than to organic factors, a complete cure is possible by Nature-cure methods, which aim at removing the cause (or causes) of the damage.

First, gradually cut out drugs of any description. It would also be better to cut out all stimulants, such as flesh foods, tobacco, strong tea and coffee, and alcohol.

The aim of treatment should be to purify and cleanse the bloodstream of all toxic substances, because, if it is clogged with these, it will corrode the heart-structures and impede their action as it passes through them on its way round the body every few seconds. Also, the thinner and clearer the blood, the easier it is for the heart to pump it. That is why too much animal-fat (butter, milk, etc.) is detrimental – it tends to thicken the blood, thus making the work of the heart harder. Powdered skim-milk, plantmilk, and yoghourt, should replace cow's milk to a great extent, and vegetable fats should replace animal-fats.

General dietary principles.

1. Replace white bread and white flour with wholewheat bread and flour. Even these should be eaten in moderation and should be partly replaced by potatoes, soya-bean flour, soya-bean milk (Granogen), and ripe bananas.
2. Replace all white sugar and white-sugar products (preserves, sweets, chocolates, etc.) with natural sugars (Barbados sugar, honey, molasses, figs, dates, sultanas, etc.).
3. Replace ordinary tea and coffee with rutin tea, or salus tea, and dandelion coffee. (See *Appendix* for source of supply.)
4. Replace alcoholic drinks with fresh fruit juices, and raw vegetable-juices. (Bottled vegetable-juices are obtainable from most health-foods shops.)
5. Replace table-salt, and other condiments, with garlic powder, kelp powder, celery powder, and Dr. Gilbert's Bio-salt.
6. Avoid rich stews, sauces, puddings, and pastry.
7. Avoid over-eating and late-night eating. Always get up from the table feeling that you could have eaten a little more. Masticate thoroughly.
8. Eat generous amounts of vegetables, conservatively cooked in a very little water, in a closed pan, with no added salt or soda. Better still, eat them raw (juiced). For this you will need a juice-press.
9. A mixed salad at the midday meal can be preceded by home-made lentil-and-vegetable soup. A jacket potato can replace bread at this meal (unless potato is going to be served at the evening meal). A mashed-up banana, with yoghourt, or a few dates, will round off the meal. A little fresh unsalted butter may be eaten with the potato or bread.

Grapes and celery are rich in substances which help to keep the heart healthy. Honey, which should entirely replace sugar and sugar-products such as jams and other preserves, is a most valuable heart-food. It is used by some doctors in Germany for patients suffering from heart troubles such as angina pectoris, coronary insufficiency, high blood-pressure, and irregular heart-beat. These doctors inject it into a vein, together with the heart-drug strophanthin, the effectiveness of which it enhances. Forest honey, gathered by wild bees, is richer in minerals than meadow honey.

Breakfast should consist of wheatgerm cereal, millet flakes, a little linseed (ground-up), together with some soaked dried-fruit such as apricots, pears, or peaches, and a spoonful of soya-bean milk. To this mixture, add a dessertspoonful of whey powder and 1 of Yestamin (brewer's yeast powder), 3 calcium and 3 Lecithin tablets (these can be ground up with the linseed in a small electric coffee-mill), 3 acerola tablets or a small teaspoonful of vitamin C powder (see *Appendix*), 1 teaspoonful of wheatgerm oil, 2 vitamin E (emulsified) capsules, a little warm water to mix, and a spoonful of plantmilk.

Elimination of toxic-wastes, through the skin, is very important. A not-too-hot bath containing about 1 lb. of common Epsom salts or 'Salus' bath-salts (see *Appendix*) should be taken twice a week, followed by skin-friction with a rough towel. (No soap should be used in the bath.) A wet (or dry) friction with a rough towel should be a daily practice. The bowels, too, should be given a wash-out with plain warm water in an enema syringe, once or twice a week, or a small dose should be taken at bedtime of powdered compound of rhubarb.

An occasional day on 'fruit-only', preceded by a heaped teaspoonful of Epsom salts in $\frac{1}{2}$ pint of hot water, helps elimination of toxic wastes, which tend to accumulate in the body and to impede the working of the heart.

Drink slowly, only if and when thirsty, and never with meals. Fruit, raw vegetable-juices, rutin or salus herb-tea, and a cup of tea containing a pinch of Epsom salts, before breakfast, should supply all the liquid you need. *This pinch of salts is most important.*

137

Sometimes, heart trouble is caused by a small bone in the spinal column being out of alignment. This presses on nerves which control the heart. This type of heart-trouble, characterized by changes in the heartbeat, can be put right by manipulation of the spine by a qualified chiropractor. (The name of one in your district can be obtained from the address given in the *Appendix*.)

Limb massage is also a great help to the heart – to some extent it can take the place of walking exercise, for very weak people. Gradually, it would be advisable to stop taking all the allopathic drugs you may have been given, and, instead, take the following homoeopathic mixture:

Tincture of Crataegus (Hawthorn)	½ oz.
Tincture of Cactus grandiflorus	½ oz.
Tincture of Convallaria	½ oz.
Capsicum	30 mins:

The dose is 5 drops, in water, before meals, 3 times daily. (This can gradually be increased to 10 drops per dose.) Take also Mag. phos. (3 pilules after meals.)

An alternative remedy is Crataegus opix., which contains Vasotonicum, made by Intermedics Ltd. of Hitchin, Herts.

Between meals, 1–2 Acerola (vitamin C) tablets should be sucked. (It is impossible to overdose with vitamin C, as any surplus of the vitamin not required by the body will be eliminated.)

Biochemic Kali. phos. should be taken at bedtime. The dose is 5 pilules. (Allow them to dissolve slowly under the tongue.)

Whenever possible, outdoor walking exercise should be taken every day, together with deep breathing as you walk. Life should be taken quietly and easily, doing everything slowly – eating slowly, drinking slowly, breathing slowly, moving slowly up steps – and resting with legs and feet supported on a high stool or chair, as often as possible.

Deep breathing helps relaxation, without which there can be no real rest or relaxation for the heart.

A heart-attack can be relieved by placing a hot (flannel) compress over the region of the heart, by taking 2 drops of spirits of camphor in a little hot water sweetened with honey (every 5 minutes, for an hour), and by inhalation of smelling-salts made of trichlorethylene crystals.

Mental and emotional upsets or strains, also over-excitement, must be avoided; so, too, must physical exertion and strenuous pursuits. All drinking water should be boiled, to get rid of the chlorine in it which destroys vitamin E. (For further reading on the subject, see *Building a Healthy Heart*, by Eric Powell, N.D., published by Health Science Press, and other books listed in 'Books for future reading'.)

Hot compresses to the spine help the heart. For this treatment, a towel about 18 inches long, folded lengthwise, is needed. It should be wrung out in very hot water, and applied lengthwise down the spine, for 2–3 minutes. Repeat the hot applications 6–7 times, and follow it with some deep kneading of the back muscles, the patient lying more on his side than his stomach.

HEPATITIS

(See 'Liver Troubles'.)

HIGH BLOOD-PRESSURE

This is usually due to hardening of the arteries whose walls lose their elasticity and become narrowed, or it can be due to an increase in the thickness of the blood. Both these changes mean that greater pressure is needed to pump the blood through the blood-vessels, and that the heart (the pump) has to work harder. It *can* be related to a shortage of magnesium in the blood.

But high blood-pressure *can* be cured (or considerably reduced) if the sufferer has sufficient strength of mind to live for a time almost exclusively on raw foods, omitting all flesh foods, all sugar (except natural sugars, such as honey, grapes, dates, etc.), and reducing the intake of starchy foods and of animal fats (butter, milk, and cream). Animal fats should be replaced by vegetable fats (nut-butter, vegetable-oil margarine) and vegetable oils (corn oil, sunflower-seed oil, soya-bean oil, wheatgerm oil, etc.).

Animal fats tend to thicken the blood. Milk, which is rich in animal fat, should be taken only in small amounts; it should be replaced by skim-milk powder, plantmilk, and soya-bean milk (Granogen), all of which contain no animal fat. Cream should be replaced by yoghourt. Pastry, cakes, puddings, etc. made with white flour, white sugar, margarine, and/or lard, should be avoided.

The chief item in the diet, however, should be vegetables, raw vegetable-juices, salads dressed with vegetable oil and cider-vinegar, and fruit, especially grapes and apples. Cheese and eggs (in moderation), soya-beans, soya-bean flour, lentils and lentil flour, nuts of all kinds, millet (seeds and flakes), sesame seeds, sunflower seeds, brewer's yeast, wheatgerm, groats (dehusked oat grains), barley-grains, etc. should take the place of flesh foods. You will, of course, need a small mill for grinding the nuts, seeds, and grains. You will also need a juice-press, for juicing your raw vegetables. Some vegetable-juices (carrots, beetroot, celery, tomatoes) are obtainable in bottles, from health-foods shops, ready for use, but green vegetable-juices are not obtainable in bottles, and so for these you will need a juice-press, as they are essential to your daily diet, especially nettle-juice, which tones the walls of the arteries. Pure bottled apple-juice, also grape-juice, is obtainable. Avoid tinned juices. Fresh fruit is better eaten whole, with its pulp, than juiced.

It is advisable at first to semi-fast for a day or two on vegetable-juices, and fruit-juices, omitting all solid food. This fasting period should be preceded by a large early-morning dose of Epsom salts, to clear the bowel of all waste-matter.

Rutin tea and dandelion coffee should replace ordinary tea and coffee. Garlic powder should replace table-salt, and salted foods (including salted butter) should be avoided. The

ing and insufficient mastication of food which, when swallowed, calls for more stomach-acid to deal with its digestion than properly-chewed food calls for; over-eating at a meal; arguments and disagreements at meal-times; and, last but not least, the indiscriminate mixing-together of foods at the same meal, irrespective of whether or not they are compatible. (See 'Compatible and Incompatible Foods'.)

Conversely, strange as it may sound, indigestion *can* be caused by an insufficiency of hydrochloric acid in the stomach. This can be due to emotional upset before, during, or after a meal, or to a lack of B vitamins, or simply to the ageing process. (Most middle-aged and elderly people suffer from slight stomach-acid deficiency.) Without sufficient hydrochloric acid in the stomach, the food you eat (especially protein) is not digested properly; its digestion is slowed up, so that it remains too long in the stomach and starts to ferment, to produce 'gas', and to cause belching. Without sufficient acid, the minerals iron and calcium are not absorbed either, and anaemia may possibly result. The deficiency can be remedied by taking brewer's yeast (rich in the B vitamins) with meals, and either a tablet of glutamic-acid hydrochloride, or 1 teaspoonful of fresh lemon-juice (or cider-vinegar) in warm water, before meals. If none of these things help, and if you still get indigestion after eating, then lack of stomach-acid is not the cause of the trouble. The cause *may* be lack of bile. The remedy for this is tincture of Golden Seal (Hydrastis), 2–3 drops in 1 tablespoonful of warm water, before meals.

Another possible cause is a deficiency of digestive-enzymes in your gastric juices. Older people often suffer from indigestion for this reason. It can be remedied by taking tablets made of dried pineapple juice (Bromelaine tablets), which is rich in digestive enzymes (see *Appendix*). Fresh pineapple, when obtainable, is even better. Outdoor exercise is also essential.

After a few days of rest and of fasting, your diet can include non-acid fresh fruits. These (grapes, sweet apples, pears, etc.) must be really ripe. Dried fruit such as apricots should be washed, then soaked overnight in water. Your diet can also include soothing drinks of Biobalm food-beverage. This contains malted slippery-elm powder which is very nourishing and soothing. Keep to this fruit and milk diet for a further day or two, then gradually build it up to include small amounts of all cleansing foods (salads, etc.) as well as raw vegetable-juices. Wholewheat home-made bread may be eaten in moderation (it should be toasted) but avoid mushy foods that need no chewing, such as cereals mushed up with milk, milk puddings, porridge, etc. Avoid also starch and sugar foods, such as cakes, puddings, pies, sweet biscuits, buns, etc. Starch and sugar mixtures cause indigestion and flatulence; so, too, do starch-sugar-and-acid-fruit mixtures, such as fruit pies, or jams and marmalade eaten with bread or puddings. Foods such as these, whose components are incompatible, *must* be avoided.

Chew all food very thoroughly, especially starchy foods such as bread, so that the saliva is thoroughly mixed with it before it is swallowed. Starch digestion begins in the mouth, with the action on the food of digestive enzymes (in the saliva). Just chewing a piece of dry bread will sometimes cure the trouble because the saliva is strongly alkaline.

Drink all liquids between meals, never *with* them. Never eat to repletion, but get up from a meal feeling that you could have eaten a little more. Allow 5 hours to elapse between meals; in fact, if you are not hungry, do not eat until you are.

Avoid strong tea and coffee, table-salt, white bread, white sugar, jams, sweets, chocolates, and all fried or greasy food. If salt is used, it should be Dr. Gilbert's Bio-salt. A little kelp powder (dried seaweed) provides not only seasoning, but is a rich source of essential minerals and trace-elements.

Always rest for a while after meals. Discomfort can often be relieved by taking 1 papain-compound tablet (see *Appendix*). The papaya juice in the tablets is rich in digestive ferments.

A good homoeopathic remedy is Nux. vomica. 3 (3 pilules before meals) especially if the indigestion is due to general debility and tiredness. If due to emotional upset, try Ignatia. 6.

INFLUENZA

You fall a victim of 'flu when you are in a low vitality state, i.e. when your system is clogged with food-residues through eating incorrectly, getting insufficient exercise, living in stuffy rooms lacking in oxygen, neglecting your bowels, etc.; also when you are emotionally disturbed, or worried.

It is essential to breathe fresh oxygenated air at all times of the day and night, because, without oxygen, the food you eat cannot be properly assimilated; this means that, unless elimination (via the bowels) of semi-assimilated foods is efficient, your bloodstream gets poisoned with bacterial toxins produced by bacteria that feed on the un-eliminated food-residues in the bowel, and a poisoned bloodstream provides an ideal breeding-ground for germs of all kinds, including the influenza virus. Germs cannot thrive and multiply in a clean bloodstream that is devoid of waste-products, because they feed only on toxic wastes.

If, however, you do fall a victim to it, you can best help your body's efforts to get rid of it by resting in bed and fasting for a few days, taking only drinks of hot lemonade or orangeade, of alpine-herb tea, and of apple-juice, all of which help elimination through the bowels and kidneys. It is better to eat no solid food, as digestion of solid food uses up vital energy, and this must be conserved as much as possible, to fight the infection.

If your body-temperature rises, stay in bed, in a warm but well-ventilated room, and do not attempt to reduce the temperature of the body by taking aspirin or any other drugs – a rise in temperature is the means whereby the body burns up, and rids itself of, rubbish and toxins in the blood, and it should, therefore, be regarded as curative.

Elimination of effete matter through the bowels must be helped by a nightly dose of either a herbal laxative (such as 'Innerclean') or of compound powdered rhubarb. An early-morning dose of Epsom salts in hot water (1 heaped teaspoonful), followed by hot drinks every 2 hours, but no solid food, should also be taken.

One of the hot drinks should be a herb tea made with equal quantities of boneset-herb, peppermint herb, and elder-flowers, plus 1 teaspoonful of composition powder. (For the recipe, see 'Herbal Recipes'.)

A concentrated essence of elderflowers, mint, and composition powder, can be obtained, ready for dilution with hot water, from most health-foods shops.

Homoeopathic pilules of Cadmium sulph. (C.M. potency), alternated with pilules of cinnamon (200 potency) should be taken in between the hot drinks. Five pilules of one or the other should be taken every 2 hours, throughout the day. They should be allowed to dissolve slowly under the tongue. Cadmium sulph. will antidote post-influenza depression, and can be continued for a week or two.

The hot drinks can be sweetened with a trickle of honey, if liked. They will produce sweating, which will help elimination of poisons through the skin. The sweat should be removed with a rough towel, and, as soon as body-temperature is normal, a hot Epsom salts bath should be taken, using a bath-brush on the skin, but no soap. The diet should consist of fresh fruit and fruit juices for a further 24 hours.

INSOMNIA

This can be due to mental or to physical causes (or both). Worry can cause tension, and an inability to relax and to give oneself up to sleep; it also causes a shortage of phosphates in the blood. This can be remedied by taking bio-chemic Kali. phos. (potassium phosphate) pilules. (Two should be taken before meals and 4 at bedtime; allow them to dissolve slowly under the tongue.) A warm bath or a hot foot-bath at bedtime is sometimes helpful. The bed should be warm, the mattress firm and even, and the bedclothes warm but light (cellular blankets are best). A small muslin bag containing lemon-thyme and dried hops, the scent of which will help to soothe and relax the nerves, can be attached to the pillow on which your head rests. After the warm bath, do not dry your body too thoroughly; to swathe it in a clean warm sheet, half-dry, may help you to sleep better.

The herbal remedy is tincture of Passiflora (passion flower). The dose is 5–6 drops. It can also be obtained in tablet form, and taken with a hot drink of herb tea at bedtime. (Lime-blossom, rosemary, hops or cowslip herbs, or a mixture of all four can be used.) It can be sweetened with honey.

JAUNDICE

See 'Liver troubles'.

LARYNGITIS

Rest the voice as much as possible. Keep to a light diet, taking hot lemon drinks with honey, and alpine-herb tea to help bowel action. Keep warm, and apply a large folded handkerchief, wrung out in cold water and vinegar (equal parts), to the front of the throat, re-wetting it every hour. Gargle with red-sage tea, made with 1 oz. of red-sage, $\frac{1}{2}$ pint of hot water, and $\frac{1}{2}$ pint of hot vinegar. Also spray the back of the throat with tincture of Hydrastis, several times a day, and take homoeopathic Hydrastis, 3 pilules every 2 hours.

The hot lemon drinks should contain 2–3 cloves, or 1 drop of oil of cloves.

LEUCORRHOEA

See 'Catarrh of the vagina'.

LEUKAEMIA (Granulocytic Leukaemia)

This has been treated with great success by Dr. Hartwell (of the National Cancer Institute at Bethesda, Maryland, U.S.A.) with an alkaloid substance related to Colchicine, which is derived from the plant Colchicum (Autumn Crocus).

Raw beetroot juice has been found by Dr. Ferenczi of Hungary to be very beneficial.

Lymphocytic leukaemia in children. This is treated with great success at the National Cancer Institute in Maryland, U.S.A., with a drug called Vincristin, which is made from Vinca rosea (periwinkle) plant.

LIVER TROUBLES

The signs of liver-congestion are abdominal fullness and discomfort, with a feeling of tenderness on the right side, under the lower ribs, and also in the stomach region. This is usually accompanied by yellowing of the complexion and of the whites of the eyes, furred whitish tongue, lack of appetite, and often by headaches, nausea (or actual vomiting of bile), diarrhoea, and depression of spirits. A bilious attack can often be averted by taking teaspoonful doses every few minutes of raw lemon juice in which a small coffee-spoonful of common salt has been mixed. (People who are subject to bilious attacks should cut down their intake of fats, eat more of the starchy foods, and never eat fats or fatty foods without some starchy food with it.)

A reputed cure for congested liver is a diet consisting entirely of grapes and nothing else (except water) for a week to 10 days. The water (previously boiled) can be flavoured with fresh lemon-juice which will help the cleansing and decongesting process. About 1½ pints per day should be drunk, and at least 2 lb. of grapes should be eaten. They should be ripe and sweet. Bottled grape-juice (obtainable from health-foods shops) may take the place of fresh grapes, but fresh grapes are preferable, and Malvern water (which is pure spring-water) is preferable to tap-water. It can be obtained from some health-foods shops, and from some wine-and-spirits shops; or distilled water can be used.

While on the water-and-grapes diet, it would be as well to take a 10-drops dose of the following mixture, in water, 2–3 times a week for the bowels; it should be taken at bedtime:

Fluid extract of Berberis	1 oz.
Fluid extract of Dandelion	1 oz.
Fluid extract of Liquorice	½ oz.
Fluid extract of Camomile	1 oz.

After 1 week to 10 days, or as soon as the symptoms have subsided somewhat, the diet can gradually be stepped-up to include vegetable juices (especially radish juice, beetroot juice, and artichoke juice, all of which are very beneficial to the liver), baked potatoes, carrots, celery, etc., but flesh-foods (meat, fish, poultry, etc.) should be excluded, and animal fats (butter, milk, etc.) cut down to a minimum.

Fresh milk should be replaced to a great extent by dried skim-milk powder, whey powder, and plantmilk. Flesh foods can be replaced by cottage-cheese, nuts, millet and sunflower seeds, wheatgerm, brewer's yeast, milk-protein (Casilan), goat's milk yoghourt, and egg-yolk (but eggs should be restricted to 3 a week). Salt and other condiments should be replaced by kelp powder, celery powder, and garlic powder. Sugar should be entirely omitted and replaced by honey and black molasses. Tea and coffee should be replaced by dandelion-herb tea and dandelion coffee with chicory. Alcoholic drinks should be replaced by grape-juice, or apple-juice. Oranges and orange-juice should be avoided, but lemon-juice in hot water is beneficial, taken every morning, before breakfast. Half a grapefruit can take its place 2–3 times a week. A homoeopathic remedy is Berberis (5 drops of the fluid extract in hot water, before meals), together with a 4-grain pill of Yellow Dock (Rumex

149

Crispus) or take Dr. Vogel's artichoke remedy, Chelicynara. (See *Appendix*.)

HEPATITIS (Inflammation of the Liver)

Only rice-water should be ingested for a few days at first. This is made with brown unpolished rice (Lima rice, like all other 'Lima' products, is organically-grown and, therefore, nutritionally rich). The rice (2 tablespoonfuls) is simmered in 2 pints of water for about 2 hours, in a covered pan, then strained, and the resulting liquid is taken in wineglassful doses every 2 hours. It should be made fresh every day. On the third or fourth day, drinks of dandelion tea may also be taken, and thereafter the diet may be of the type prescribed for liver troubles.

There is a herbal remedy that contains several herbs, including greater celandine, dandelion, and berberis. It is called 'Hepata' (see *Appendix*); or take Dr. Vogel's Chelicynara 3 times daily. For torpid liver, take Hydrastis 30 (Golden Seal) or Chelidonium majus 3 (Celandine).

JAUNDICE

This calls for the help of a doctor. Until he comes, take nothing to eat or drink except fresh lemon juice, diluted with water (a few sips every 15 minutes).

A fast of 2–3 days is usually advised, although some doctors allow yoghourt to be eaten in small amounts. They advise a nightly warm-water enema, to clear the bowels. The homoeopathic remedy is Chelidonium 1, or Berberis 1.

LOCOMOTOR ATAXIA

This is a spinal complaint, which can be greatly helped by physiotherapy, by Pyonex treatment (see *Some Unusual Methods of Healing* by Leslie Korth, D.O.), and by taking homoeopathic Hypericum 30 (5 pilules night and morning).

LUMBAGO

The quickest way to cure this is to stay in bed, keeping to a light diet, with frequent drinks of hot elderflower-and-mint tea (sweetened with honey, not sugar) to promote sweating. Local treatment of the painful area with heat in the form of hot-water bottles, or hot poultices made of bran or linseed-meal (or a cantharides plaster) should be given. Massage with warm Olbas oil can also be given. Internal remedies include biochemic Ferrum. phos. (2 pilules every 3 hours), also homoeopathic berberis 2x. and Rhus. tox. 4x., taken alternately (10–15 drops every 3 hours). This means that one or other of the three remedies is taken every hour. At bedtime, ½ teaspoonful of powdered rhubarb-compound should be taken, plus a hot drink of the elderflower tea, to ensure complete evacuation of the bowels next day.

MASTITIS

For this, take homoeopathic Conium maculatum 30 (5 pilules at bedtime and on rising). Apply Acacia powder, made into a thick paste with warm water, to the breast. This is harmless to a breast-fed infant.

MENIER'S DISEASE

This is a kind of migraine of the ear, caused by vaso-motor spasm. The spasm causes constriction of the blood-vessel, resulting in giddiness, nausea, and ringing in the ears, followed by dilation of the blood-vessel, which results in an accumulation of fluid in the inner ear and consequent headache and general malaise. The cause of the vaso-spasm is usually a lack of vitamin B in the diet, especially of *vitamin B.3* (Nicotinic acid), very often due to eating too much sugar. It can be remedied by omitting *all* sugar (except pure honey) from the diet, by reducing the consumption of starchy clogging foods such as white bread, white-flour cakes, biscuits, etc., and of animal fats, and by taking

151

brewer's yeast (rich in all the B vitamins), wheatgerm cereal, and wheatgerm oil ($\frac{1}{2}$ teaspoonful a day). It can be relieved by daily doses of homoeopathic Hypericum 30.

MENOPAUSE

See 'Change of Life'.

MENSTRUATION (Profuse)

A tea made of Vinca-major herb is helpful.

MENTAL AND EMOTIONAL IMBALANCE

See 'Psychosomatic diseases'.

MIGRAINE

This is the result of a vaso-spasm (spasm of a blood-vessel) causing visual disturbances, followed by vaso-dilation (enlargement of the blood-vessel), which causes an increased flow of blood to the brain, with consequent severe headache. The vaso-spasm can be remedied by diet-reform (see 'Menier's disease'), and relieved by taking homoeopathic Cyclamen (see *Appendix*).

Other possible causes of migraine are as follows:

1. An unclean toxic state of the blood, due to faulty feeding and to incomplete elimination of waste-products. These products, circulating in the bloodstream, produce irritation of the brain-tissues, and consequent headache.
2. Thickenings and congestion in the muscles at the back of the neck. These thickenings cause pressure on the vessels and nerves passing to and from the brain, with consequent headache.
3. Stress and strain of all kinds, including emotional stress, over-work, and over-play. People who drive themselves

relentlessly – who are unable to stop short of exhaustion – often suffer from migraine; they feel compelled to finish whatever they are doing, no matter how great the effort needed. They should learn to stop short of exhaustion, to take life more easily, to worry less, and to do things in a more leisurely manner. They are usually perfectionists, and, for this reason, their own worst enemies.

4. A diet deficient in vitamins (especially B vitamins), minerals, trace-elements, and possibly protein. A diet of whole, unprocessed, unrefined foods, supplemented by brewer's yeast, wheatgerm, rose-hips, and kelp tablets should be eaten.

5. Too much speeding in everything; insufficient relaxation of the brain and body; too little sleep, perhaps; excesses of all kinds; too much excitement; menstruation (which to many women is a stress and strain); all these things deplete the body's nervous energy and may trigger off an attack of migraine.

6. Certain foods can trigger off an attack in people who are allergic to these foods. Such foods include chocolate, cheese, eggs, cow's milk, tomatoes, oranges, strawberries, bananas, oats, oysters, salmon, and many others. By using the 'pulse test', you can find out which of the foods you eat is causing the allergy. Anything that, when eaten, quickens the pulse unduly is 'suspect'. (See the chapter on 'Allergies' in Linda Clark's book *Get well naturally*, published by Devin Adair, New York.)

Treatment. At the first signs of an attack (with or without visual disturbances), do not *suddenly* slump, letting go completely, but let go gradually; try to keep going as long as possible. A cup of strong (decaffeinated) coffee helps. Put your feet in hot water and apply a hot sponge or towel to the anus (bowel exit). Apply a cold compress soaked in spirits of camphor to the back of the neck, and insert a little menthol ointment into the nostrils. All these little activities will prevent you from slumping too suddenly, which causes a rise in blood-pressure and a dilation of the blood-vessels in the head, with consequent pain and pressure, and digestive disturbances.

A good homoeopathic remedy made by Intermedics Ltd. is a combination of the following ingredients:

> Cyclamen 3x.
> Gelsemium 4x.
> Iris versicolor 3x.
> Melilotus 3x.
> Primula veris 3x. (cowslip)

The dose is 10 drops, every ½ hour, till relieved.

The quickest way to rid the body of the toxins in the blood, which cause the trouble, is to fast on alkaline (vegetable) juices for a day or two every 3–4 weeks. While fasting, a warm water enema should be used daily, or a purging dose of Epsom salts taken each morning, on waking.

MULTIPLE SCLEROSIS

This is the commonest disease of the nervous system. Its symptoms come and go, so it is very difficult to diagnose in the early stages. A deficiency of linoleic acid in the blood is one of the chief causes, and this can be rectified by including in the daily diet 1–2 spoonfuls of sunflower-seed (or safflower-seed) oil. (For further information concerning diet, etc., see 'Disseminated Sclerosis'.)

NETTLERASH (Urticaria)

This is a fairly common complaint, which may be caused by eating a particular food to which the eater is allergic. Among the foods which cause nettlerash (in some people) are eggs, shell-fish, veal, pork, oatmeal, honey, strawberries, oranges, etc. Having found out, by a process of trial and error, which of the many foods you eat may be the cause of the trouble, it will be necessary to omit that particular food permanently from your diet. If this does not cure the trouble, try eating foods rich in calcium, such as apples, raw cabbage, nettles, yoghourt, buttermilk, etc., because nettlerash *can* be due to a lack of calcium in the blood. Also, take three Calcium-Plus tablets a day.

An acute attack of nettlerash should be treated as follows: Fast for 24 hours, taking no solid food, but drink frequent cups of nettle tea, flavoured with fresh lemon-juice and sweetened with a little honey. Eat apples, or drink apple-juice. Have an Epsom salts bath at bedtime, followed by a dose of Innerclean herbs, with a drink of apple juice. Apply Calendula (marigold) ointment to the affected area of the skin.

If fresh nettles are unobtainable, take nettles in homoeo-pathic form, Urtica Urens 3x. The dose is 3 pilules every 2 hours.

The remedy prescribed by orthodox medicine is an anti-histamine drug, or adrenaline.

The early symptoms of Hodgkin's disease (itching of the skin) closely resembles those of Urticaria.

NEURALGIA AND NEURITIS

Both these complaints may be largely due to a lack of calcium in the blood, so the remedy is to eat foods rich in calcium, such as raw apples, raw cabbage, nettles, yoghourt, buttermilk, cheese, almonds, etc. and to take 'Calcium-Plus' tablets (see *Appendix*). Eating apples for breakfast and nothing else – not even a drink – has been known to cure neuritis. If chewing is difficult, the apples can be grated, or pulped in a mincer or a blender, because they are better eaten raw. A pinch of bicarbonate of potash in a little hot water should be taken at bedtime and on rising. For the pain, take homoeopathic Aconite 3 (5 pilules every hour), and apply a flannel bag, filled with hot bran or linseed meal or camomile flowers, to the painful area. A hot foot-bath may also help. If heat makes the pain worse, do not apply hot bags; take frequent sips of hot water in which Ferrum phos. and Mag. phos. pilules are dissolved (5 of each). (See 'Facial Neuralgia'.)

Tic doloreux (facial neuritis). In addition to the above, sufferers could try a course of Acupuncture treatment. (See *Some Unusual Methods of Healing*, by Leslie Korth, D.O., published by Health Science Press.) A homoeopathic remedy is Gelsemium 4x. (10 drops every 2 hours). Vitamin B.12 (1 tablet per day) should also be taken.

Facial neuralgia. A homoeopathic remedy is Rhus. tox. 4x. alternating with Gelsemium 4x. (Take also vitamin B.12 – 1 tablet per day.)

Intercostal neuralgia. A homoeopathic remedy is Bryonia 3x.

Nightmare. For this, the remedy is paeony tea, made as follows: Pour ½ pint of boiling water over ½ oz. of paeony root (powdered). Stir and allow to infuse for 10–15 minutes. Drink hot, with a little honey added (also milk if liked), at bedtime. Paeony root is obtainable from Potters Herbal Supplies Ltd. (see *Appendix*).

NOISES IN THE EARS

The commonest causes are wax in the ear-holes, blockage of the Eustacian tubes due to a cold, over-dosing with aspirin, and high blood-pressure. If the noises persist, the ears should be examined by an ear-nose-and-throat specialist.

NOSE-BLEED

Pinch the lower ends of the nostrils together, breathe through the mouth, and apply a cold compress to the back and sides of the neck. Place 4 powdered-up pilules of Ferrum phos. on the tongue, and powder up 4 more, putting this powder on to two bits of cotton-wool and inserting them into the nostrils. If this does not stop the bleeding, plug the nostrils with cotton-wool or ribbon-gauze soaked in perchlor. of iron. (Always keep this home-made remedy handy.) Stretch both arms up above the head, if possible. Take 2 Ferrum phos. pilules 3 times a day, before meals, for several weeks, also homoeopathic Phosphorus 6x. (4 pilules at bedtime). Bioflavoid capsules (for vitamins C and B) would help to strengthen the walls of the tiny blood-vessels inside the nose.

NEURASTHENIA

This is another name for nervous exhaustion. The treatment is complete rest in bed for a few days (or longer, according to the severity of symptoms), in a warm but well-ventilated room. The diet should be light, nourishing, and cleansing. It should include the following: fresh fruit, sun-dried apricots, yoghourt, sunflower seeds, sesame seeds, wheatgerm cereal, kelp tablets dissolved in a little hot water and added to raw celery and other vegetable juices; cooked vegetables (potatoes should be cooked in their skins); salads; grape-juice; egg-yolk; cottage cheese; wholewheat bread or toast; honey in place of sugar and sugar-products; wild thyme tea made with cold (not hot) water; dandelion coffee; soya-bean powder (Granogen); ripe bananas; malted slippery-elm food-beverage at bedtime; and lemon juice in $\frac{1}{2}$ pint of hot water, on waking, in the morning. The following food-supplements should be added to the wheatgerm cereal and the ground-up sunflower seeds and sesame seeds: 2 vitamin E capsules, 1–4 teaspoonfuls of brewer's yeast powder, 2 acerola tablets, 2 Dolomite tablets, 2 'Calcium-Plus' tablets, and 1 vitamin B.12 tablet. (The tablets can be ground up with the seeds.) A teaspoonful of Bionektarin should be taken after each meal (see *Appendix*).

The biochemic remedy Kali. phos. will help sleeplessness. Take 5 pilules dry on the tongue, at bedtime, after your drink of slippery elm. A hot foot-bath is also helpful. During the daytime, take Calc. phos. (2 pilules, between meals). If you are troubled with neuralgia or other pain, take 2 Mag. phos. pilules every $\frac{1}{2}$ hour until relieved. If possible, a warm bath, followed by skin-friction with a rough towel, and deep breathing exercises, should be taken daily.

Homoeopathic Nux. Vomica 3x. (5 pilules before meals) could be given a trial for a few weeks. It is excellent for tiredness, debility, and nervous exhaustion.

PHARYNGITIS (Chronic Catarrh of the Throat)

Take 10–15 drops, 3 times daily, of Ammon. brom. obtainable from Inter-Medics Ltd. (see *Appendix*).

NASO-PHARYNGITIS

Obtain Eupatorium opix from the above suppliers, and take 10–15 drops, 3 times a day.

PHLEBITIS

This is an inflammatory condition of a deep vein (or veins), usually the large vein in the leg, and its branches. It is often associated with injury by injections. Although this can trigger off the trouble, the underlying cause is a highly toxic bloodstream, and only complete cleansing of the blood, by fasting and bowel wash-outs (or purging), can cure the trouble permanently.

The sufferer should stay in bed and fast on fresh-pressed

juices only, for 2–5 days, according to the severity of the condition. During these few days, a warm-water enema should be used every night, and a purging dose of Epsom salts taken next morning for the first 2 days, because it is essential to thoroughly cleanse the bowels of all effete matter.

The affected leg should be raised on pillows above the level of the rest of the body, and several times a day a small towel, wrung out in hot water, should be applied to the affected part for 2 minutes, then re-heated and re-applied (about a dozen times in all), finishing off with an ice cold application for 1 minute.

After 2–5 days, the inflammation should show signs of subsiding, and the patient can then go on to an all-fruit diet for a further 2–3 days. A hot Epsom salts bath, using 1 lb. of common Epsom salts to half a bathful of fairly warm water, can then replace the daily bed-bath. The all-fruit diet can gradually be supplemented by other foods of a plain and simple nature, i.e. by vegetables, vegetable-juices, and salads. Flesh foods should be eaten only 2–3 times a week and are better omitted altogether and replaced by eggs, cheese, milk, soya-bean milk, wheatgerm, nuts, seeds, and lentils. White bread and white-flour products, white sugar and white-sugar products, also strong tea, coffee, and condiments (including salt) should be replaced by wholewheat bread, Barbados sugar, honey, English herb-tea, dandelion coffee, kelp powder, and garlic powder.

Further 2-day fasts on an all-fruit diet, at monthly intervals, may be necessary for some people, depending upon progress. The bi-weekly Epsom salts bath, and the daily dry (or wet) friction-bath, should be continued indefinitely – it is most important.

Other helpful practices are simple deep-breathing exercises in fresh air, gentle walking exercise as soon as possible, and resting with legs raised, as often as possible. The local heat applications can be continued too, but they should always be followed by a cold application of 1 minute's duration.

All drugs, including anti-coagulants and all injections, should be refused if permanent cure by the above natural methods is desired.

Vitamin E takes the place of anti-coagulant drugs and is much safer. These drugs tamper with the blood's ability to clot, and may cause serious trouble.

One vitamin E capsule (containing 100 units of the vitamin) should be taken every day at a meal that includes a little vegetable oil. After a week, unless the blood-pressure is higher than normal, increase the dose to 2 capsules, and after 2 weeks increase it to 3 capsules, but not if the blood-pressure is higher than normal; in this case, keep to 1 capsule a day.

The biochemic remedy is Ferrum. phos. 3x., alternated with Calc. fluor. 6x. The dose is 3 pilules of one or the other, every 4 hours, between meals.

PLEURISY

The aim of treatment should be to rest the entire system, to encourage the elimination of toxins, to relieve pain, and to build up vital energy, so that the patient's resistance to infection and his powers of self-healing are strengthened. This calls for complete rest in bed, on a diet of fruit-juices and water only, for a few days (i.e. till the temperature is normal). Distention of the stomach with solid food tends to make the pain worse.

The herbal remedy is tea made with nettles, dried elderflowers, peppermint herb, and pleurisy-root. Use the recipe for nettle tea given in the Appendix. Pleurisy-root and elderflower tea is made as follows: Simmer ½ oz. of crushed pleurisy-root, ½ oz. elderflowers, and ¼ oz. peppermint, in a pint of water for about 30 minutes. Strain and add the resulting liquid to the nettle tea. Add a good pinch of ginger, sweeten with honey, and take a wineglassful (hot) frequently. Drinks of alpine-herb tea may also be taken, to help bowel action (see *Appendix*).

Apply a hot cloth, wrung out of another lot of hot nettle tea, to the painful area; cover with a dry cloth and a hot-water bottle. When the wet cloth has gone cold, remove it, gently massage the area with warm olive oil, then apply a fresh hot cloth soaked in nettle tea, and repeat doing this at regular intervals of, say, ½ hour. Alternatively, a hot linseed-meal poultice can be applied; this retains its heat longer, so need not be changed so often.

A dose of herbal laxative such as Innerclean herbs should be taken at night, or, if the pain allows, a warm-water enema should be given. As soon as the pain has subsided a little, a bath may be taken.

When the temperature is normal, a little milk can be added to the diet, also some vegetable broth, raw vegetable juices, and a baked potato. Continue this fruit-and-vegetable diet for a few days, then gradually introduce other foods such as wholewheat bread (toasted), eggs, cottage cheese, soya-bean milk, etc. Continue the nettle tea with honey, and the lemon juice in hot water before breakfast.

Homoeopathic Aconitum 3x. and Bryonia 3x., taken alternately every 2 hours, will help to bring down the temperature to normal.

PREGNANCY (Toxaemia of)

The commonest cause of still-born babies is the mother's 'deficiency' diet. Through eating over-refined foods (white bread, white sugar, etc.) her diet will lack iron and folic acid (and probably many other vitamins and minerals), and this causes not only anaemia and general weakness (so that labour and birth are more painful and difficult) but also toxaemia. This – toxaemia of pregnancy – is a very common complication of child-bearing, and can be dangerous for the mother, and fatal for the child. She may be given pills containing folic acid and iron at her ante-natal clinic, but it is preferable to obtain these vitally important substances from natural whole foods, such as green leafy vegetables (especially broccoli, spinach, endive, lettuce), wholewheat bread, salads, etc. rather than from pills. As its name implies, folic acid is found chiefly in foliage (i.e. green leaves), which is best eaten raw. (It can be juiced in a juice-press.)

Dried liver tablets are very rich in iron and in all the B group of vitamins, including folic acid, vitamin B.6 and vitamin B.12. Vegetarian mothers can substitute brewer's yeast (powdered) and vitamin B.12 tablets in place of the dried liver. Brewer's yeast is rich in all the B vitamins (except B.12) and in iron and many other essential substances. Oil of bitter almonds (2 drops in a little water) will relieve early-morning sickness.

PROLAPSED UTERUS (Dropped Womb)

This is usually the result of carrying a heavy baby in the womb, and/or of difficult labour. It can be greatly relieved by doing exercises to strengthen the internal abominal muscles (a physiotherapist will show you how to do these), and by taking biochemic Calc. fluor. (Take 3 pilules 3 times a day.) A supporting rubber ring inside the vagina is not recommended.

PROSTATITIS

This is usually caused by a faulty chemical state of the blood, which gives rise to an imbalance of the glands of the body, including the prostrate gland. The faulty chemical state of the blood can be due to one of several causes, the chief of which are excessive smoking, constipation, and a deficiency diet. A diet of white bread, white sugar, meat, boiled vegetables, fried foods, tea, coffee, alcohol, etc., is a deficiency diet. In addition, the blood could be poisoned by hundreds of chemicals used in and on our foods, and by any remedial drug that may have been taken.

The deficiency diet must be replaced by a balanced one,

composed of foods in their natural state which have not been contaminated by chemicals. Such foods *are* obtainable at all health-foods shops.

But first, a body cleansing is essential, in order to rid the blood of toxins, which are the underlying cause of the congestion, swelling, and inflammation of the gland.

For the first 2 days of treatment, only liquids in the form of diluted vegetable juices should be taken – no solid food at all. They should be sipped slowly, a little at a time, about every hour throughout the day. Apples (and apple-juice) are beneficial, but citrus fruits should be avoided. The juices and the apples can be alternated with drinks of parsley tea and dandelion tea. At night, a cup of alpine-herb tea should be taken, and in the morning a purging dose of Epsom salts in hot water (a heaped teaspoonful to $\frac{1}{2}$ pint of water). This will purge the bowels of toxic matter. It may not be necessary to repeat the dose next day, but a pinch of the salts should in future be taken in hot water every morning. This will not be sufficient to act as a purge, but will supply the body's special need for magnesium. Dolomite tablets (rich in calcium and magnesium) should also be taken, and these (and the pinch of Epsom salts) should be continued indefinitely.

The 2-day fast can be broken on the third day by eating a bowlful of vegetable broth every 3–4 hours. The broth should be made with vegetables of all kinds, cut up and stewed gently for an hour or so, including parsley and dandelion leaves (fresh if available), carrots, celery, and onions. Apples, or drinks of freshly-pressed apple-juice or grapes, may also be taken.

During these 3 days, signs that the body is making efforts to cleanse itself may appear, e.g. headache, dizziness, coated tongue, nasty taste, diarrhoea, mild sweating, etc. All these symptoms are a part of the body's natural cleansing process and they should be welcomed. They mean that the energy that would normally be used up in the digestion and assimilation of food has been utilized in removing unwanted toxins from the body. A warm bath, followed by friction of the skin with a rough towel, should be taken daily, as the skin is a most important factor in the elimination of toxins.

On the third and fourth day of treatment, the diet should be on the following lines:

On rising	A pinch of Epsom salts in a hot drink.
Breakfast	A sweet ripe apple or some grapes.
11 a.m.	A drink of hot vegetable broth.
Lunch	A pear or an apple.
4 p.m.	A drink of vegetable broth.
Evening meal	Another drink of vegetable broth or of raw carrot juice.
On retiring	An apple, or apple-juice, or grape-juice.

This diet may with great benefit be continued for a further day. It is essential that, for these first four or five days, no tea (other than herb or dandelion tea) and no coffee (other than dandelion coffee) should be taken.

During the following week, the meals should be on the following lines:

Breakfast	Apples, or any fresh fruit in season; a little yoghourt.
11 a.m.	Hot vegetable broth, or fresh raw tomato juice, or raw vegetable juices, including beetroot tops, carrots, parsley, celery, etc.
Lunch	A raw salad (dressed with sunflower-seed oil) consisting of grated raw carrot, lettuce, watercress, parsley (chopped), tomato, onion, dandelion leaves, accompanied by a piece of mild cheese, cottage cheese, or cream cheese, one slice of wholewheat bread, and unsalted butter. Follow with soaked dried apricots and yoghourt.
4 p.m.	A cup of herb tea or dandelion coffee, with milk and honey.

Evening meal Any three vegetables, cooked in a covered pan without salt or soda, in a little boiling water. The water in which they are cooked should be drunk before eating them; it can be flavoured and made more beneficial by the addition of a little 'Vecon' (vegetable-concentrate). The vegetables should be mashed, a little soya-bean oil added, and then a sprinkling of chopped parsley. A potato cooked in its skin should be included.

This fruit and vegetable diet should continue for a further week if there is still any discomfort or pain, but, as soon as these symptoms decrease, more protein in the form of eggs, cheese, nuts and seeds (especially sunflower seeds and pumpkin seeds), soya beans, lentils, wheatgerm, brewer's yeast, etc., should be added gradually to the diet. Flesh foods are not necessary and should be omitted; so also should sugar and sugar-products, tea, coffee, alcoholic drinks, mineral waters, condiments, salts, and pickles. Kelp powder and vegetable salt (Herbamare), should replace table-salt. Salad dressing should be made with sunflower-seed oil and cider-vinegar (equal quantities), and honey can replace sugar.

Sunflower seeds and pumpkin seeds are especially beneficial because, in addition to Zinc, they contain trace-elements and active ingredients, which stimulate the production of prostatic hormones, and thus help to restore the hormonal balance of the gland, which has been upset.

Wholewheat bread and flour should replace white bread and white flour; cow's milk should be cut down to a minimum; it can be replaced by plantmilk and soya-bean milk. Such things as cakes, pastry, and puddings should be avoided. Dandelion coffee should replace ordinary coffee.

Local treatment should include hot hip-baths, which should be followed by a splash of cold water on the gland area. Congestion can also be greatly reduced by the application (to the gland area) of a T-shaped cold compress. It should be applied after the hot hip-bath, just before retiring at night, and kept on all night. The T-compress is made of two pieces of clean sheeting. One of the pieces (about 14 inches wide) is wrapped round the abdomen; the other piece (about 7 inches wide) is passed between the legs and pinned to the front and back of the abdominal piece. Both pieces should be wrung out in cold water before applying. A pair of trunks should be worn over the compress.

Deep massage and finger pressure should be given daily to the backs of the heels, i.e. round both sides of the Achilles tendons and the surrounding tissues.

Special remedies. Homoeopathic tincture of Sabal berries (5–10 drops) should be taken in a little water, 3 times a day, after meals. Combined with the blood-purifying Echinacea herb, it is included in a preparation called 'Urgenin' (see *Appendix*). Other important remedies that should be taken are:

Dolomite tablets (3 per day) for Magnesium
Bonemeal or Calcium-plus tablets (3 per day)
Kelp tablets (3 per day, in vegetable juices)
Vitamin E capsules (2 per day, with wheatgerm cereal)
Yestamin (Brewer's yeast powder) 1–4 teaspoonfuls with wheatgerm cereal.
Kali. phos. (3 pilules before meals)

For the pain. Take homoeopathic Sulphur 6 oz. in alternation with Rhus. tox. 30.

PSORIASIS

If you eat meat, it should be boiled for 5–10 minutes before cooking in the usual way, to extract the taurine in it. Taurine is one of the unimportant amino-acids in animal-protein, and some people, due probably to a metabolic defect in their ability to produce a particular enzyme, are unable to deal with it properly, and it causes psoriasis. Meat-eaters with such a metabolic defect cannot be cured of their complaint, but, so long as they stick to their special diet, the complaint can be kept under control. Diabetes is another example of a complaint, due to a metabolic defect, which can be controlled by diet.

Unfortunately, boiling removes not only taurine from the flesh-foods but important minerals and water-soluble vitamins. There must also be a great loss of minerals and vitamins through the sufferer's skin, which flakes off from his body in great quantities. These lost minerals and vitamins must be replaced by adding vitamin and mineral supplements to the daily diet. To replace lost B vitamins, he should take wheatgerm cereal, a little wheatgerm oil, dried-liver tablets (or, if a vegetarian, brewer's yeast daily, and 1 vitamin B.12 tablet 3 times a week). Rose-hip or acerola tablets should be taken to replace vitamin C; bonemeal (or calcium-plus) and dolomite tablets to replace lost minerals, and kelp tablets to replace lost trace-elements. Kelp tablets can be crushed and taken in raw vegetable-juices.

Treatment should start with a short 2-day fast, taking only drinks of fresh fruit juices; or vegetable juices, diluted with a little water, every 2–3 hours. The bowels should be washed out with a warm-water enema at night, and next morning a teaspoonful dose of Epsom salts should be taken in $\frac{1}{2}$ pint of hot water, before any other drink. This cleansing of the bowels of all effete matter is most important.

This should be followed by a hot bath, in which about 1 lb. of common Epsom salts is dissolved, and the skin frictioned with a bathbrush (except on the inflamed area). No soap should be used. The friction will stimulate circulation and help elimination of poisons through the skin. After the bath, olive oil should be applied to the inflamed areas, gently smoothing it in. Sometimes, Rumex ointment, or medicinal clay (Claydos), moistened, and applied to the bad patches, is helpful (see the *Appendix*); so, too, is natural or artificial sunlight, a gradually-acquired sun-tan being the best external remedy.

After the 2-day fast, the diet should consist of fruit for a further 2–3 days. It can include ripe bananas (mashed up) eaten with yoghourt or soya-bean milk (Granogen); grapes, apples, pears, oranges, and grapefruit; also sun-dried apricots, peaches, figs and prunes.

Following the few days on fruit and yoghourt, other natural whole foods should gradually be added, one by one. These can include whole-wheat bread, unsalted butter, a little farmhouse or cottage cheese, green salads (dressed with sunflower-seed oil or corn oil, and cider-vinegar), potatoes cooked in their skins, green vegetables, especially nettles (when available), raw vegetable-juices, especially nettle-juice, watercress juice, celery juice, and carrot juice. (See 'Juices' in *Appendix*.)

Flesh foods are best excluded from the diet; they should be replaced by nuts of all kinds, soya beans, soya-bean powder (Granogen), lentils, millet seed, sunflower seed, sesame seed, wheatgerm; by cheese, eggs, and milk-protein (Casilan). Garlic powder and celery powder should be used instead of table-salt, honey instead of sugar for *all* sweetening, honey or malt-extract instead of jams and preserves, and dandelion coffee instead of ordinary coffee.

A 5-day 'all-fruit' diet should be repeated at regular intervals, or whenever the symptoms become more troublesome than usual.

To help bowel regularity and to cleanse the blood, take homoeopathic Sulphur 30x. (2 pilules 3 times a day, between meals). Biochemic Nat. mur. 3x. should replace it after a few days, and should be continued indefinitely, unless a great deal of raw green leafy vegetables and salads (especially watercress and celery) are eaten every day.

Sarsaparilla was the 'wonder' remedy of bygone days – and still is, if taken regularly every day for several months.

PSYCHOSOMATIC DISEASES AND MENTAL DISORDERS

Psychosomatic diseases, which are physical illnesses caused by a disturbed mind, are the result of conflict between a part of the brain called the cortex, which is the controlling part, and a part called the Di-encephalon (the brain-stem), which is the instinctive and oldest part – the part that, in primitive man, developed first.

In animals, the two parts (the cortex and the stem) work in close co-operation, but in Man, whose cortex is far more developed than the cortex of an animal's brain, this close co-operation between the two parts no longer exists.

The brain-stem's instinctive reactions to fear seem senseless and unintelligent to the cortex of Man's brain. For example, a man looking at a fierce roaring lion in a cage is instinctively frightened, and the instinctive part of his brain (the stem) prepares his body for flight. But although the controlling reasoning part (the cortex) knows that this instinctive fear is unnecessary because there are strong iron bars between him and the lion, the instinctive part (the stem) knows nothing of such artificial things as bars – it (the stem) still reacts to the presence of the lion as it did in primitive times – i.e. as if no bars existed. These normal fear-reactions of the brain-stem annoy and alarm the cortex, and this cortical alarm is flashed back to the stem, causing it to react by even intenser preparation for flight. Thus, a vicious circle is set up, and psychosomatic disease is the result. The form it takes varies in various people – some get skin symptoms, others get circulatory and blood symptoms, others get nervous complaints. All of them are caused by conflict between the two parts of the brain.

Take another example: A physically-poor specimen of a man may have an instinctive fear of his bigger and more powerful co-worker in business or factory, but this fear is suppressed, because the reasoning part of his brain (the cortex) tells him that his co-worker will do him no harm physically. His instinctive fear is converted by the reasoning

169

part of his brain (the cortex) into an emotion, such as dislike of his job, or jealousy of the colleague, or a hope that he (the colleague) will die. Such an emotion, however, is never allowed to become a conscious one; it is suppressed, and the suppression of it results in conflict between the instinctive and the reasoning parts of his brain. This mental conflict reacts upon his physical body, causing bodily disturbances and symptoms of ill-health, because mind and body are inseparably inter-related and inter-dependent. The conflict can be resolved, and the symptoms of ill-health cured, only by examining the suppressed emotion in the cold light of reason. In this way it can be converted from a destructive harmful emotion into a constructive one, having no harmful effect on physical health. But to do this, critical self-analysis and self-understanding is needed, and most people are incapable of this without the help of a psycho-analyst; he helps them to detect their suppressed thoughts and emotions.

Quite often, a disturbed state of mind, bordering on insanity (with or without depression, suicidal tendencies, fatigue, apathy, restlessness, and irritability), is entirely due to mineral and vitamin deficiencies, and to a low blood-sugar level of the blood, caused by eating a deficiency diet and too much sugar. This sounds contradictory – if you eat a lot of sugar you would think it would raise the blood-sugar level in the blood, but it does not work that way. If the pancreas is healthy and able to secrete plenty of insulin, an excessive amount of sugar in the blood is neutralized by the insulin to such an extent that the excess becomes a deficiency, causing the blood-sugar level to fall well below normal, and this leads to the mental, emotional, and physical disturbances mentioned above. It also leads to moral imbalance and criminal tendencies. (See *Body, Mind, and Sugar,* by Dr. E. M. Abrahamson and A. W. Pezet, published by Holt and Co.)

Regarding mineral deficiencies, a lack of the mineral magnesium, for example, can give rise not only to some of the above disturbances, but also to mental confusion and disorientation, to hallucinations, to convulsions, to nerve-tremors and muscle-twitchings, to irritability, exhaustion, hysteria, an inability to think straight, and to mental instability bordering on insanity.

A lack of magnesium is also related to heart troubles of all kinds; to diseases of the nervous system; and to irregularity of the heart-beat. This is because, without magnesium, calcium (which regulates the heart-beat) cannot be properly utilized. A lack of magnesium is also related to kidney disease, to high blood-pressure, to enlargement of the prostate-gland, to calcium absorption and the de-mineralization of bone, and to many other physical disturbances.

The remedy for mineral deficiencies (including magnesium deficiency) is a diet consisting of natural, whole, unprocessed foods (eaten raw as far as possible), including fresh vegetables and salads, wholewheat bread (there is no magnesium in white bread or white flour), raw nuts and seeds, etc. In addition, vitamin B.12 and bonemeal tablets (rich in calcium, phosphorus, and magnesium) should be taken (bonemeal can be replaced for vegetarians by dolomite tablets and 'Calcium-Plus' tablets). Kelp (seaweed) tablets should also be taken, for often there is an iodine shortage, and consequent thyroid-gland malfunction.

It is certain that, if patients in mental hospitals were correctly fed on whole, natural, unrefined, unprocessed foods, instead of on the usual over-refined, processed, chemicalized, over-cooked foods, and if all white sugar and white-sugar products were excluded, mental hospitals would be half empty, and the need for them would gradually disappear.

Dr. Graupner of Munich, Germany, author of *Adventures in Healing*, tells how hundreds of depressed and mentally-ill people, some with suicidal tendencies, have been helped by homoeopathic doses of Tincture of Hypericin, a substance derived from the plant Hypericum (St. Johns Wort), plus irradiation of the whole body with ultra-violet light (sunlight).

But mental instability and depression sometimes have to

be treated by 'shock' treatment; this brings the patient 'down-to-earth', so to speak. Of the three types of shock-treatment in use, only electric shock-treatment is now used.

Another curative plant used extensively in American mental hospitals is an Indian plant called Rauwolfia. It has taken the place of shock-treatment for wildly disturbed, violent patients. It is also used for patients with high blood-pressure. It can be obtained in tablet form (see *Appendix*).

PYORRHOEA

This is an inflammatory condition of the gums, accompanied by a constant discharge of pus into the mouth. It is a constitutional ailment, due to years of wrong feeding, and too much mushy food, which gives the jaws no exercise. It can usually be cured, in time, by correcting the diet, including in it foods that need well chewing. There is no need to have all your teeth extracted unless the poison from them is making you feel very ill.

White bread and white flour products should be replaced by wholewheat bread and flour. White sugar should be entirely eliminated from the diet; brown Barbados sugar or honey should replace it.

Start by having a 'fruit-only' diet for 2–3 days, and a daily enema (or a herbal laxative) to cleanse the bowel of poisons. Rinse out the mouth 2–3 times a day with water to which ½ teaspoonful of tincture of myrrh has been added. Also massage the gums night and morning with your finger and thumb dipped in pure lemon juice, or Eucalyptus oil, or tincture of Hydrastis.

After the initial 3-day 'fruit only' diet, the subsequent diet should include the following: plenty of salads consisting of watercress, lettuce, onions, shredded cabbage, etc.; ripe fruits especially apples, oranges, lemons. Instead of meat, wheatgerm cereal, soya beans, lentils, milk, yoghourt, buttermilk, nuts and seeds should be eaten.

Elimination of poisons through the skin must be helped by

daily wet or dry skin-friction (with a hot Epsom salts bath 2–3 times a week). Exercise in the fresh air is essential every day. It is most important, too, that there should be a proper evacuation of the bowels every day. If the bowels are sluggish, a herbal laxative such as 'Innerclean', or 'Natex 12' (see *Appendix*), should be taken at night, and a warm-water enema used once or twice a week.

QUINSY

Pour 1 pint of boiling water on ½ oz. of composition powder, 12 cloves, and 1 oz. of red sage. Cover. When cold, strain, and add the juice of 1 lemon, and use hot, as a gargle, some of which should be swallowed.

Gargle also with tincture of Hydrastis (a few drops in ½ cup of warm water) and take Homoeopathic Baryta. carb. 6x. and Belladonna. 3, alternately, every hour, for 2–3 days. (See 'Tonsilitis'.)

RHEUMATISM

The term rheumatism covers a wide range of aches and pains, chiefly in the muscles and joints of the body. It is more often than not due to faulty feeding habits – i.e. to the eating of 'deficiency' foods, of too much acid-forming food, and too little alkaline-forming food. Lack of exercise, with consequent incomplete elimination of the body's waste-products due to sluggish bowel, kidney, and skin action, is a contributory cause. It can also be brought on by mental or emotional strain, because this disturbs the nice acid-alkaline balance of the blood, increasing its acidity. In order to right this imbalance, the blood, as it journeys round the body, deposits surplus acid in the joints and muscles. This causes swelling, the swollen tissues press on nerve-endings, and pain is the result.

First and foremost, therefore, it is important to avoid acid-forming foods (starches, sugar, and flesh foods), also incompatible foods (see page 204), to eat plenty of alkaline-forming foods (fresh-picked vegetables and salads, eaten raw as far as possible); to encourage the elimination of waste-products from the body via the bowels, kidneys, and skin, not only by correct feeding, and drinking of cleansing (herbal) teas, and raw vegetable-juices, but also by exercise (with deep breathing) to promote sweating (if possible). What to do if exercising is too painful will be described after details of diet have been given.

Self-treatment should start with a short 2–3 day fast, taking only raw alkaline juices (carrot, celery, parsley, potato and nettle) diluted with a little Malvern water, and drinks of mixed-herbs tea, sweetened with a little honey. The herbs should include dried nettles, Burdock root, and rosemary, using a tablespoonful of each to 1 pint of boiling water, adding 1 tablespoonful of maté tea (obtainable from health-foods shops) and of alpine-herb tea (see *Appendix*). At bed-time, a dose of fluid extract of rhubarb (30 drops) should be taken in a little water, and next morning 1 heaped teaspoon-ful of Epsom salts in ½ pint of hot water. This and the rhubarb should purge the bowels of all effete matter. (30 drops equals ½ teaspoonful. 1 teaspoonful may be needed by some people who are normally constipated.)

Repeat the dose of Epsom salts next morning. (A bowel wash-out with a warm-water enema may be used instead of the salts, if preferred.) It is essential that the body should have a thorough spring-clean of this sort if it is to derive benefit from subsequent diet-reform. The bedtime dose of rhubarb should be taken once or twice a week for several weeks, or until bowel action becomes easy and regular and there is what feels like a complete evacuation every day. Extract of rhubarb is made from the roots of the plant (it is the stems that are stewed and eaten, but they should not be eaten by rheumatics). The extract is not only a gentle laxa-tive, but it also gives tone to the musculature of the bowel, and is anti-rheumatic. It can be taken in powder form, if preferred (½–1 teaspoonful).

After the short 2–3 day fast, little drinks of barley-water, made at home with natural brown pot-barley, should be taken with a little milk, 3–4 times a day. To each cupful, add 1 teaspoonful of acacia powder and 1 teaspoonful of slippery-elm powder, mixed to a smooth paste with a little warm water before adding to the barley-water. This drink, with a little pure honey, is a complete meal. Yoghourt made of goat's milk (obtainable at most health-foods shops) together with a few sun-dried apricots (soaked overnight, but not cooked nor sweetened) may also be taken.

After a further 2–3 days, the following foods can be gradually included in the diet: fresh fruit (apples, pears, melon, grapes, pineapple) avoiding oranges, lemons, rhubarb, plums, damsons, and all fruits ending in 'berry', like strawberry, raspberry, etc.; vegetables (juiced raw, also lightly cooked), potatoes cooked in their skins, salads (to include dandelion leaves, garlic, onions, and parsley) dressed with soya-bean oil and cider-vinegar; a little wholewheat bread (toasted), unsalted butter, farmhouse or cottage cheese, lightly-cooked egg (not fried), but no flesh foods. Cakes, pastry, biscuits (except Ryvita or oatcakes), tarts, pies, jams, sweets, and chocolate, tinned foods, table-salt, pickles, condiments, sauces, and alcohol, should also be omitted.

All tap water should be boiled before drinking, and is better replaced by Malvern water, which is pure spring-water, free of all impurities. This can be obtained from most health-foods shops, also from some wine-and-spirits shops. Filters for filtering rain-water (which is considered best of all by T. Hartley-Hennessy, author of *Healing by Water*), can be bought from Harrods of London.

No aluminium cooking or storage vessels, or teapots, should be used.

Exercise in the fresh air every day, taking deep breaths, if only for 10–15 minutes, is very important. If this is not possible (because too painful), massage of the limbs and back, together with deep breathing practice and assisted movements, should replace it. A daily all-over friction of the body should be given with a rough brown linen towel, and a hot bath containing about 1 lb. of Epsom salts should be taken twice a week. No soap should be used. It should be followed by a rub-down with a rough friction towel, to stimulate excretion of poisons and acids through the pores of the skin.

The painful parts can be massaged with warmed olive oil, or Olbas oil (see *Appendix*). Painful joints can be treated with pure lemon-juice, applied neat.

Special remedies include the following food-supplements, biochemic and homoeopathic remedies: Dolomite tablets (3 a day), for calcium and magnesium (two minerals which rheumatics often lack); a small teaspoonful of wheatgerm oil; Yestamin (brewer's yeast powder, 1–4 teaspoonfuls) on wheatgerm cereal; kelp tablets (3–4 dissolved in vegetable water together with a little celery powder and garlic powder); acerola or rose-hip tablets (1 to be sucked every 3–4 hours); alpine-herb tea (see *Appendix*); maté tea; fluid extract of dandelion (30 drops) and Urtica Urens 6x. (10 drops) in a cup of dandelion coffee, once or twice a day; biochemic Nat. phos. 6x. (2 pilules before meals) and biochemic Silica 6x. (2 pilules after meals); a pinch of Glaubers salts (Nat. sulph.) in early-morning tea or hot water; biochemic Mag. phos. 6x. for the pain (5 pilules dissolved in a spoonful of hot water, and sipped as often as required); biochemic Kali. mur. 6x. (5 pilules at bedtime, dissolved under the tongue); homoeopathic fluid-extract of rhubarb (30 drops), or powdered rhubarb-root ($\frac{1}{2}$ teaspoonful mixed with a little molasses, taken with a few sips of hot water, 2–3 times a week, at bedtime). For pain eased by movement, take Rhus. tox. 3. (5 pilules before meals). For pain eased by rest, take Bryonia. 3. (5 pilules before meals).

For gouty rheumatism with sore and aching feet, homoeopathic mother-tincture of Ledum is helpful. (The dose is 5 drops in 1 tablespoonful of water, 3 times a day, between meals.)

SHINGLES

The underlying cause of this ailment is the chicken-pox virus which can lie dormant in the body for many years. In youth or middle-age, the ailment is not a serious one, but it *can* be serious in older people. It becomes active as a result of bowel toxaemia due to constipation and the eating of too much flesh foods.

The diet should, therefore, exclude all flesh foods. It should include plenty of vegetables, raw vegetable-juices, salads, and fresh fruit (see 'Constipation').

Treatment. Eat nothing solid for 2 days, but drink orange-juice, apple-juice, and nettle tea made with fresh or dried nettles (for recipe, see page 199). The bowels should be given a warm-water wash-out each night whilst fasting, followed by a hot Epsom salts bath. A teaspoonful dose of Epsom salts should be taken early next morning, in $\frac{1}{2}$ pint of hot water. A 3-day 'all-fruit' diet should follow the short fast, then gradually a more normal but completely meat-free diet can be taken. Massive doses of vitamin B.12, are needed. One 25 microgram tablet should be taken with each meal.

To the affected parts of the skin, apply moistened slippery-elm powder, and cover with clean linen or muslin. If this does not bring relief, try using a little olive oil. An alternative is to bathe the affected skin-area with vinegar and warm water (equal parts).

The herbal remedy is Hydrastis (Golden Seal). The dose is one tablet or 5 drops of the fluid extract in a little hot water before meals, 3 times daily.

A homoeopathic remedy is Urtica urens 6x. (nettles), alternated with Ranunculus 2x. and Anacardium 4x. The dose is 3 pilules of Urtica urens at mid-morning, 3 pilules of Ranunculus at mid-afternoon, and 3 pilules of Anacardium after tea. If in pain and unable to sleep, take Zincum Valerianicum 4x. (3 pilules) at bedtime, and again later, if necessary.

SINUS TROUBLE

This is not an ailment; it is a symptom of a 'deficiency' diet – a diet lacking in fresh raw foods including salads, raw vegetable juices, and fruit. The consumption of milk and of other animal protein, also of starch and sugar foods, should be drastically reduced. All salt and salted foods, also all sugar (except honey, and dried fruits rich in natural sugar) should be omitted. The following food-supplements should be taken every day:

Four 'Calcium-plus' tablets (these contain vitamin D). They can be milled with your nuts and seeds, and eaten with wheatgerm cereal, mashed bananas, and a tablespoonful of soya-bean powder (Granogen), or plantmilk (cow's milk should be avoided). Acerola or rose-hip tablets can be eaten as often (and with as much enjoyment) as sweets or chocolates, which, of course, must also be avoided. Dried brewer's yeast powder (Yestamin) should be sprinkled over the nuts and cereal. (Start with 1 teaspoonful, gradually increasing to 4.) This, and wholewheat bread, will provide all the necessary B vitamins (except B.12), so a 10 microgram B.12 tablet should be taken every other day. Unsalted butter (in moderation) should be eaten, and sunflower-seed oil used instead of cooking-fats. Kelp tablets (3–4) should be dissolved in a little hot water (or vegetable-water) and, together with a little garlic powder and a little 'Vecon', added to vegetable-juices or vegetable soups.

Needless to say, outdoor (daily) exercise, with deep breathing, is essential.

SKIN TROUBLES

These are not usually diseases of the skin itself, but are the result of the throwing-off of blood-impurities by the Life-force of the body. The fact that perspiration is poisonous is proof of the truth of this statement.

It is most important that skin trouble should be treated

from within – never suppressed by the external application of lotions, ointments, etc. If treated externally by strong lotions, ointments, etc., the trouble will be driven inwards, and will sooner or later manifest itself as asthma, bronchitis, kidney disease, or some other ailment, in an attempt to find an outlet. For skin troubles are Nature's efforts to throw out impurities from the body, and therefore the best way to treat them is to work *with* Nature, i.e. to encourage elimination of impurities through the skin, by cleansing washes, by sunbaths, and by a salt-free diet in which some vegetable oil, vegetables, and vegetable-juices, salads, and herbal teas, are included. The following are especially beneficial: watercress, nettles, dandelion, burdock-root tea, camomile tea, comfrey-herb tea, sarsaparilla root. Make a decoction with the following herbs: 1 oz. sarsaparilla root, 1 oz. Yellow-dock root, 1 oz. Burdock root, $\frac{1}{2}$ oz. Poke-root. Stew the herbs gently in 1 quart of water till reduced to 1 pint. Sieve, allow to cool. Dose: 1 tablespoonful after meals. To help bowel cleansing take powdered rhubarb ($\frac{1}{2}$ teaspoonful in 1 teaspoonful of molasses or honey) with a hot drink at bedtime. For scurviness, redness, and pustules, moisten and rub with your own saliva.

For eczemas caused by bacteria, for boils, for infected wounds and sores, for suppurating acne, the use of Usnic acid ointment is advised. (Usnic acid is made from beard-lichen.) Homoeopathic Rumex ointment is equally good. Neither of them is suppressive. Some wheatgerm oil should be taken. Only a vegetable-oil (or slippery-elm) soap should be used.

For ringworm, castor-oil applied externally is the remedy. To moisten with saliva is also curative. The diet should include 1 teaspoonful of wheatgerm oil (or other vegetable oil) every day. This can be mixed with 1 teaspoonful of cider-vinegar, and put on salads. Garlic and kelp powder should replace table-salt.

179

Skin-cancer. Podophyllin, an extract from the American Mandrake plant Podophyllum, has been used with great success by Dr. Hartwell of the National Cancer Institute, U.S.A.

Slipped disc. Many sufferers have been cured by Pyonex (pus-expelling) treatment, probably because the trouble may sometimes be due not to pressure of a displaced cartilage, but to the exudative products of the original injury. Pyonex treatment relieves the congested state in the region of the disc, causing a drainage of purulent matter through the pores of the skin. Blistering, cauterization, mustard plasters, liniments, etc. all act in the same way, but far less effectively. (See *Some Unusual Methods of Healing*, by Leslie Korth, D.O., Health Science Press.)

Sore throat. A thick piece of toast soaked in hot vinegar, wrapped in a handkerchief, should be applied and bandaged on. Renew the poultice every 2 hours. Gargle with hot sage-tea and vinegar, or with Hydrastis (a few drops of the tincture in warm water), and take hot lemon drinks with honey, or teaspoon doses of glycerine-lemon-and-honey mixture.

SORE TONGUE

This can be due to over-acidity of the stomach. To remedy this, fast for 24 hours, taking only alkaline drinks such as raw carrot-juice, potato-juice, and little drinks of slippery-elm food-beverage. To ease the soreness, chew a piece of raw onion, working it well in, wherever the tongue is sore. Also use a tincture of myrrh mouthwash (a teaspoonful in a glass of warm water) and swallow some of it.

Soreness of the whole mouth, points to a shortage of B vitamins; to remedy this, eat wheatgerm, also brewer's yeast.

STERILITY

This is often due to a lack of vitamin E in the diet, and can be remedied by eating wholewheat bread, wheatgerm cereal, wheatgerm oil, nuts and seeds, and by taking 2–3 vitamin E capsules daily. Eliminate (or cut down) cigarette smoking.

STONE IN THE KIDNEY OR BLADDER

See 'Bladder and Kidney Troubles'.

STYE ON THE EYE

If persistent, styes are usually a sign of general debility and of a toxic state of the blood, although they *can* be aggravated by eye-strain. Treatment should aim at purification of the blood by means of diet-reform, herbal blood-purifiers (see page 63), and efficient elimination of waste-products from the body. This means that the bowels and skin should be kept active, taking a natural vegetable laxative, such as 'Innerfresh'. If the bowels are costive, take plenty of exercise in the fresh air, and a hot Epsom salts bath once or twice a week. The eyes should be bathed with a lotion made of eyebright herb. Apply a touch of golden-eye ointment to the stye, or it can be rubbed with a gold ring moistened with saliva. A homoeopathic remedy is Belladonna 3. (4 pilules every 2 hours till the stye comes to a head and bursts; then Hepar sulph. 6x. every 2 hours).

SWELLING OF FEET OR ANKLES, OR LEGS

For this, take the herbal tea recommended for Dropsy. If worse early in the day it is due to kidney dysfunction, if worse at night, it is due to heart weakness.

SYNOVITIS OF THE KNEE

The pain can be eased by drinking hot elderflower and mint tea frequently, by bathing the knee with the hot tea, finishing off by applying to it a cloth wrung out in the hot liquid, securing it in place with a bandage. Take biochemic Ferrum phos. pilules, alternately with Silica pilules, every 2 hours. Resting the leg as much as possible also helps healing.

TEETHING TROUBLES

Put 2 pilules of homoeopathic chamomile into the feeding bottle, 3 times a day.

TOOTHACHE

Plug the offending tooth and massage the gum with oil of cloves, or hold neat brandy in the mouth.

TONSILLITIS

Treatment should aim at ridding the system of the cause of the trouble (toxins in the system), as well as relief of the symptoms by means of gargles, etc. Tonsils are detoxicating organs; they enlarge and get inflamed only when the blood is overloaded with toxins which it cannot get rid of through the normal channels of elimination – (the bowels, kidneys, and skin). Tonsillitis is usually associated with, and the result of, constipation. Treatment should include either warm-water bowel wash-outs or a few doses of a natural vegetable laxative such as 'Innerclean' herbs or powdered rhubarb-root. Hot Epsom salts baths will help elimination of poisons through the skin. For the first day or two, keep to a diet of fresh fruit only, with hot drinks of elderflower and mint tea, sweetened with honey. If there is fever, no solid food should be taken until the temperature is normal – only fruit, fruit-juices, vegetable-juices (carrot, etc.) and tea made with St. Johns Wort (Hypericum) herb.

The throat should be gargled with neat lemon-juice, a little of which can, and should, be swallowed. Once or twice a day it should be sprayed with tincture of Hydrastis. For this, an atomiser spray can be bought from any good chemist. A piece of toast, soaked in hot vinegar and wrapped in a folded handkerchief, can be applied to the front of the throat over the tonsil area, and bandaged on. A dose of tincture of Echinacea (10 drops in a little water) should be taken during the daytime, every 4 hours. At bedtime, a cold vinegar-compress should be applied and bandaged on.

The tonsils are valuable organs of selective elimination. The fact that they become inflamed is a direct result of a toxic state of the blood, which can be righted by correcting the diet, by breathing exercises, by regular outdoor exercise, and by homoeopathic medicine. They should not be removed surgically unless a bacteriological examination of them, made when the acute inflammation has subsided, shows that they are diseased and exuding pus. Even in this case, homoeopathic remedies should be tried before surgical removal is decided upon.

These remedies include Phytolacca 3. (4 pilules before meals), Drosera 3. (4 pilules after meals), and Kali. mur. night and morning. The Hydrastis throat-spray should be used regularly, and, above all, the diet should be corrected, and there should be complete evacuation of the bowels every day. (See 'Adenoids and Tonsils'.)

TUBERCULOSIS OF THE LUNGS

This can be cured if tackled in the early stages. Diet is all-important; so too is an abundance of rest and sleep in rooms with permanently open windows, gentle daily exercise and deep breathing in the fresh air, and daily cleansing of the body in a warm bath. Warm sea-water baths are very beneficial. If real sea-water baths are unobtainable, add about

½ pound of Tidman's sea-salt to a ½ bathful of comfortably warm water at home. Sea-salt (especially prepared for the table) should be used instead of table-salt, for seasoning. Ideally, the sufferer should live near the sea, or in a high dry mountainous region.

A warm-water enema, to wash out the bowels, should be given a few times at the start of treatment. Subsequently, the inclusion of laxative foods such as soaked prunes, figs, apricots, molasses, honey, wholewheat bread, bran, together with vegetables, fruits, etc., in a properly-balanced daily diet, should ensure thorough bowel evacuation every day.

In most other ailments, treatment starts with fasting for a few days on natural juices, but the patient with T.B. lungs is not fasted, nor is he encouraged to eat a preponderance of alkaline-forming foods. These foods (vegetables, vegetable-juices, fruit, salads, etc.) should, of course, be eaten, but the following acid-forming foods should also be eaten; home-made wholewheat bread; farmhouse cheese; free-range new-laid eggs; raw nuts, seeds and cereals, including almonds, millet-seed, sesame-seed, sunflower-seed, linseed, groats, barley-flakes, etc. These should be ground-up in a small nut-mill or coffee-mill and mixed with wheatgerm cereal. All-bran, powdered fenugreek seeds, milk protein (Casilan), whey powder, soya-bean powder (Granogen), and powdered brewer's yeast (Yestamin). A porridge-plateful of the mixture, moistened with a little warm water and eaten with raw farm-fresh milk (unpasteurized if possible), should be eaten every day. Milk still warm from the cow is the ideal sort, but difficult to obtain unless you live on, or near, a farm.

Fenugreek seeds are nutritionally of great importance, being very similar in composition to cod liver oil, which to some extent they can replace. They are obtainable in powder-form (see *Appendix*). Cod liver oil in malt should be taken, in small doses, after meals, and a garlic oil capsule with meals.

Other important items in the daily diet are calcium-rich foods such as goat's milk yoghourt; raw vegetable-juices especially cabbage-juice, turnip-tops, kale, and broccoli; also whey powder, raw milk, cheese, almonds, sesame seeds, millet-seed, soya-bean milk and soya-bean flour.

Raw, fermented vegetable-juices (carrot, beetroot, celery, and tomato), obtainable from health-foods shops, also fermented wheatgrains (see *Appendix*), are rich in ferments which seize and kill the tubercle bacilli. However, unfermented juices (especially beetroot and watercress) are also very beneficial, and $\frac{1}{4}$ cupful of them should be taken every day, preferably about 10 minutes before a meal, together with 2–3 alfalfa tablets, 3 kelp tablets, and a small teaspoonful of Vecon. Take fermented juice before one meal, the unfermented before the other meal.

Flesh foods are neither necessary nor advisable. If they *are* eaten, salmon, halibut, herrings, liver, and kidney, are nutritionally the best. Drinks should include frequent sips of slightly-warmed farm-fresh cow's milk or goat's milk (unpasteurized, if possible); tea made with nettles and nettle-seeds; tea made with Iceland moss; tea made with comfrey-root; alpine-herb tea; apple-juice, and grape-juice. Dandelion coffee should replace ordinary coffee. Other drinks include fresh-pressed orange juice or lemon juice, starting the day with the juice of half a lemon in hot water and ending it with apple-juice, or a raw sweet apple, at bedtime. Drinks should be taken between meals, never *with* them. Honey or molasses should be used for sweetening, not sugar. Milk jellies made with warmed (not boiled) milk, Gelozone (Irish Moss), and pure honey, are nutritious and delicious if flavoured with fresh fruit-juice. Salted foods should be avoided, including salted butter.

A remedy to ease coughing and to assist expectoration is made as follows: Slice up a raw onion on a porridge plate, cover with honey. Leave overnight. Take sips of the juice, as required. A preparation called 'Liquifruta', which is similar, using garlic juice and sea-onion, can be bought from most chemists.

Biochemic Calcium phos. 6x. should be taken daily

(2 pilules between meals), and, if there are night-sweats, Ferrum. phos. (5 pilules at bedtime).

ULCERS ON THE TONGUE

Take biochemic Silica 6x. The dose is 3 pilules, before meals, and at bedtime. (See 'Sore Tongue'.)

URAEMIA

This is due to defective function of the kidneys, causing an excess of urea and of other waste-products in the blood. A 'mono' diet of bananas only, for a week or longer, eating at least half a dozen a day, is advised. (See 'Bladder and Kidney Troubles'.)

VARICOSE VEINS

These are dilated veins, and can appear on any part of the body, but they are most often seen on the legs. When they occur in the rectum, they are called haemorrhoids, the common name for which is 'piles'.

The following are some of the more usual causes:

1. A sluggish circulation of the blood. This is often due to lack of exercise.
2. Constipation. This is usually due to wrong diet, lack of exercise, and a sluggish liver.
3. Over-weight and/or too much standing. These are causes in so far as they can trigger off the trouble, but they are not basic causes. However, they should be treated – over-weight, by a reducing diet, together with calcium tablets and kelp tablets; too much standing, by sitting down whenever possible, and by resting in the body-slant position whenever the opportunity occurs. This position – a

position in which the feet and legs are raised and supported on something higher than the head and trunk – reverses the pull of gravity on the body-fluids. It assists the circulation, and relieves the work of the heart.

Neither surgical operation nor injection-treatment cures the trouble – indeed, injections can be dangerous. Cure lies in removing the causes, not in just relieving the symptoms.

Treatment should, therefore, be constitutional as well as local. A most important part of it is daily outdoor exercise – preferably a brisk walk, to speed up the circulation of the blood and to stimulate the liver. Also rest, with the legs in the body-slant position. Trunk-bending-and-twisting exercises, in the fresh air or in any airy room, stimulate the liver, and, therefore, are also helpful.

Treatment should commence with a short fast, on juices only, for 24–48 hours, preceded by a purging dose of Epsom salts (a heaped teaspoonful in $\frac{1}{2}$ pint of hot water). This dose should be repeated and doubled next morning if the previous day's dose did not purge the bowels, because it is absolutely essential that the accumulation of waste-products and toxic substances in the bowel should be got rid of.

After the 2-day fast, the diet for the next 7–10 days should be plain and simple, consisting chiefly of fresh (and dried) fruit, salads, vegetables (cooked *and* raw), raw vegetable-juices, and yoghourt. At the end of this time (but not until then), a little wholewheat home-made bread, a little unsalted butter, and a little cottage-cheese may be added to the diet; but flesh foods, also sugar, salt, and salted foods, should be avoided. Honey should replace sugar for all sweetening purposes, and kelp powder should replace table-salt.

Further periods on an all-fruit diet for two or three days may be necessary from time to time, depending upon what improvement takes place.

Local treatment. This should include a daily wet (or dry) friction of the whole body with a rough towel, and twice a week a fairly warm Epsom salts bath (using no soap), followed by cold sponging of the affected leg. Comfrey leaves or a loose bandage, dipped in cold comfrey-herb tea (for recipe see page 198), should be applied and left on all night. An elastic stocking should be worn during the daytime. The lower end of the mattress should be raised by placing rolled-up blankets under it, at the foot-end of the bed. Thus, while you sleep, your feet and legs will be slightly elevated, and this will assist circulation.

Special remedies.

One vitamin E capsule with meals, 3 times a day.
Biochemic Calc. fluor. 6x. – 5 pilules at night. Biochemic Ferrum. phos. 6x. – 5 pilules mid-morning.

Dr. Gilbert's biochemic remedy (V.122) can replace the Calc. fluor. and the Ferrum. phos. The herbal remedy is Dr. Vogel's Hyperisan, which contains the herb Hypericum (see *Appendix*).

VARICOSE ULCERS

Great benefit has been obtained from a medicinal clay called Claydos (see *Appendix*). It is mixed to a paste with hot water and applied (on lint) to the ulcer. The clay removes and absorbs the toxins from the ulcer and its surroundings. Powdered comfrey-root can be used instead of Claydos; so, too, can warm mashed carrots, spread on lint, because carrots are rich in vitamin A.

For long-standing septic ulcers, a homoeopathic remedy is Pyrogen. A few globules are dissolved in an 8 oz. bottle of distilled water and 1 tablespoonful of the mixture is taken once a day. Ionic medication, using Zinc, is often helpful.

VOICE (Loss of)
See 'Laryngitis'.

WARTS

Anoint with oil of sulphur or with fresh elderberry juice, 2–3 times a day. Warts (and other growths such as polypi, fibroid tumours, cysts, etc.) can be the long-term result of vaccination, and the remedy for this is homoeopathic Thuja 200. One dose a week, for 1–2 weeks, will suffice. Biochemic Silica 6x. should also be taken, not only for warts but for lumps and growths of all kinds, and foods rich in vitamin A eaten daily. These include carrots, tomatoes, kale, broccoli and other greens, egg-yolk, cheese, and halibut-liver oil.

WENS

These are small growths, about the size of a pea, on the scalp. They are harmless, and should be left untouched. Graphites ointment or castor oil will soften them, and they may then disappear, by dispersing.

Graphites tablets can be taken, but this is not necessary unless the growth(s) get larger.

WHITLOWS

The homoeopathic remedy is Hepar. sulph. 3x. 3 times a day, with biochemic Silica 3. at bedtime and on rising. Hot bread-poultices, or hot fomentations of slippery-elm powder mixed with boiling water, help to relieve pain and swelling.

WHOOPING COUGH

The patient must be kept in a warm but well-ventilated room, isolated from other people. The diet should be light and easily-digested, avoiding milk and milky foods. In fact, the best diet for the first week or 10 days consists of fruit and/or vegetable juices or vegetable soups, omitting all solid food.

The distressing cough can be relieved by little drinks of linseed tea (for the recipe, see page 199), and by massage of the chest and back with Olbas oil or camphorated oil. Spread Oil of Garlic (or chopped garlic bulbs) over two pieces of plain white lint, which have been cut to the shape of the patient's feet. Apply them so that the lint (not the oil) is next to the skin, which should first be vaselined. Place oiled silk under the lint, and bandage into place.

WORMS

People troubled with worms (usually children) should eat ground pumpkin seeds and raw carrots, in milk, for breakfast on 2–3 consecutive mornings, after which no food of any kind should be eaten until the next morning, when breakfast should again consist of the pumpkin seeds and grated carrots. Two hours later, a purging dose of Epsom salts should be taken, followed by a hot drink. If the worms do not come away in the copious stools which the salts should cause, the same breakfast should be repeated next day, preceded by a fast, and followed by another purging dose of salts. If the worms still do not come away, an enema containing an infusion of Quassia (1 oz. to 1 pint of boiled, cooled water) should then be given, and garlic oil (3 capsules) taken at bedtime.

APPENDIX

Health-foods, food-supplements, remedial products, and treatments are obtainable at the following addresses:

Herbs, herbal-teas, herbal remedies, etc.

Carter Bros., Glen Laboratories, Shipley, Yorks.
Potters Herbal Supplies Ltd., Douglas Works, Wigan, Lancs.
Frank Roberts, The Herbal Dispensaries, Forest Edge, Hanham, Bristol.
The Society of Herbalists, 21 Bruton Street, London W.1.

Dr. Bach's Flower Remedies

The Bach Healing Centre, Sotwell, Wallingford, Berks.
Most homoeopathic chemists.

Biochemic remedies

The Biochemic Centre, Church Trees, Grantham, Lincs.
Carter Bros., Glen Laboratories, Shipley, Yorks.
Chromo-biochemic Co., 2 Harrington Drive, Nottingham.

Acupuncture

The name of the nearest practitioner can be obtained from The Acupuncture Association, 2 Harrowby Court, Seymour Street, London W.1.

Biochemic treatment

Dr. Peter Gilbert, 42 Harley Street, London W.1.
Mr. Eric Powell, N.D., 21 Bloomfield Road, Harpenden, Herts.
Dr. Gilbert's Biochemic Laboratories, Grantham, Lincs.

Appendix

Chiropractic treatment

The name and address of the nearest practitioner can be obtained from The British Chiropractors Association, 120 Wigmore Street, London W.1.

Homoeopathic treatment

The Nature-cure Clinic, 13 Oldbury Place, London W.1. (also from private practitioners)

Homoeopathic remedies

Inter-Medics Ltd., Portmill Lane, Hitchin, Herts.
E. Gould and Son, 67 Moorgate, London E.C.2.
A. Nelson and Son, 73 Duke Street, London W.1.

Nature-cure

The British Naturopathic Training College, Netherhall Gardens, London N.W.3.
The Hospital of Natural Healing, Sprowston Road, Forest Hill, London S.E.22.
The Nature-cure Clinic, 13 Oldbury Place, London W.1.
The Society of Herbalists, 21 Bruton Street, London W.1.
(also from private practitioners. See advertisements in *Health for All*)

Osteopathic treatment

The British School of Osteopathy, 16 Buckingham Gate, London S.W.1.
The Nature-cure Clinic, 13 Oldbury Place, London, W1.
The Osteopathic Clinic, 25 Dorset Square, London N.W.1. (also privately)

Pyonex treatment

Leslie Korth, D.O., 159 St. John's Road, Tunbridge Wells, Kent.

Short-wave treatment (for arthritis, cancer, diabetes, goitre, multiple sclerosis, etc.)

Dr. Jules Samuels, Plantage Parklan 20, Amsterdam, Holland.

Mr. Brookes, N.D., Prestow, Gubbols Road, Bomen Heath, Shrewsbury, Salop.

A list of practising members of the British Naturopathic and Osteopathic Association can be obtained from the Association's headquarters at 6 Netherhall Gardens, London N.W.3. Residential naturopathic establishments include Enton Hall, near Godalming in Surrey; Tyringham House, at Newport Pagnell in Buckinghamshire; Champneys, at Tring, in Hertfordshire; and Weymouth Hydro at Weymouth, in Dorset. Many others advertise in *Health for All*, and *Here's Health* magazines.

Health Foods. The following natural whole foods are obtainable from most health-foods shops, including The London Health Centre, 78 Baker Street, London, and 'Wholefood', 112 Baker Street, London. The 'health-foods' departments of some of the bigger London stores also sell them:

Wholegrain cereals (wholewheat flour, rye flour, oatmeal, barleyflour, lentil flour, soya-bean flour), wheatgerm cereal, barley kernels, barley-germ (Gestaal), dried skim-milk powder, soya-bean milk powder (Granogen), Casilan, plant-milk, nut butter, nut creams, nuts and seeds including sesame seed, sunflower seed, pumpkin seed, millet seed, buckwheat seed; vegetable oils (cold-pressed), vegetable-oil margarine (sunflower-seed, safflower, and corn oil); unsalted butter, cottage cheese, goat's milk yoghourt; natural brown (Barbados) sugar, preserves made with natural brown sugar, chocolate made with brown sugar; sun-dried fruit including apricots, peaches, pears, prunes, figs, dates, sultanas, and tree-ripened bananas; bottled raw vegetable-juices, apple-

juice, grape-juice; Malvern water; honey-marmalade, honey
(English and imported); black treacle, crude black molasses;
Gelozone (Irish Moss) for making jellies; Vecon (vegetable
concentrate); dried herbs (Chiltern herb-farm); Dr. Gilbert's
bio-salt; sea-salt; celery powder; garlic powder, and kelp
powder (Lusty's); Yestamin (brewer's yeast); English herb-
tea, dandelion tea, maté tea, alpine-herb tea, Mu tea,
Ginseng tea (a Lima Health Foods product), dandelion
coffee.

Food-supplements and Remedial Products (*Makers of*)

Healthcrafts Ltd., 81 High Street, Godalming, Surrey.
Hofel's Pure Foods Ltd., Woolpit, Bury St. Edmunds,
Suffolk.
W. Lusty and Co., Westcliff on Sea, Essex.
LIMA Health Products, Station Road, Winchmore Hill,
London N.21.
Organic Vitamin Co., Potten End, Berkhamsted, Herts.
Potter's Herbal Supplies Ltd., Douglas Works, Wigan,
Lancs.
Rayner and Pennycook Ltd., Rayvit House, Govett Ave.,
Shepperton, Middx.
Modern Health Products, Davis Road, Chessington,
Surrey.
Dr. Gilbert's Health Foods, The Biochemic Centre,
Grantham, Lincs.
Swiss Health Products, Blackburn Road, Wheelton,
Chorley, Lancs.

Supplements (in tablet or capsule form) include the following:

Acerola (vitamin C), Alfalfa, calcium-plus, dolomite,
bonemeal, dried liver, kelp, Bio-flora, Florus (powdered),
rose-hip, vitamin E, vitamin B.12, wheatgerm oil.
Most of them are obtainable from health-foods shops.

Remedial Product	*Supplied by*
Alpine herb tea (for constipation)	Potter's Herbal Supplies. Also most health-foods shops.
Agar-agar (powder)	Mapletons Health Foods, Garston, Liverpool 19. (Also some health-foods shops.)
Agiolax (laxative) (Psyllum Seeds)	Inter-Medics Ltd., Portmill Lane, Hitchin, Herts.
Antifect tablets	Potter's Herbal Supplies.
Antitis	Potter's Herbal Supplies.
Acacia Powder	Potter's Herbal Supplies.
Biobalm Food-beverage	Modern Health Products, Davis Road, Chessington, Surrey. (Stocked by most health-foods shops.)
Biral (daytime sedative)	Inter-Medics Ltd.
Bioflavonoid capsules	Organic Vitamin Co.
Bio-nektarin	Inter-Medics Ltd.
Bromelaine (pineapple) tablets	Organic Vitamin Co.
Carob-bean powder	Rayner & Pennycook, Rayvit House, Govett Avenue, Shepperton, Middx.
Casilan milk-protein	Most good chemists.
Calcium-plus tablets	Healthcrafts Ltd.
Curophyll herb-tea	Potter's Herbal Supplies.
Cyclamen opix. (for migraine	Inter-Medics Ltd.
Chelicynara	Swiss Health Products.
Circulinol	G. R. Lane, Gloucester.
Claydos medicinal clay	G. Ashley & Co., 104 Christchurch Road, London S.W.2.
Composition powder	Potter's Herbal Supplies.
Comfrey herb	Potter's Herbal Supplies.
Comfrey root powder	Potter's Herbal Supplies.

195

Remedial Product	*Supplied by*
Cinnamon powder	Potter's Herbal Supplies.
Cucumber (powdered)	Hofel's Ltd., 121 Bengeo Street, Hertford.
Dandelion (Fluid Extract of)	Potter's Herbal Supplies.
Dandelion Coffee	Hofel's Pure Foods Ltd.
Enpac (Acidophyllus milk) for colitis	Boots, Chemists.
Eastons Syrup	Any good chemist.
Educol (for constipation)	Modern Health Products.
Eyebright (Euphrasia herb)	Potter's Herbal Supplies.
English Herb-tea	Health-foods Shops.
Elderflower and Mint (Fluid Extract of)	Potter's Herbal Supplies. (Also most health-foods shops.)
Enzygest tablets	Healthcrafts Ltd.
Fenugreek Seeds (powdered)	Potter's Herbal Supplies.
Fermented Wheat-grains	E. L. David (Biologist), 6 Redcliffe Close, London S.W.5.
Florus	Healthcrafts Ltd.
Four Oils (for external massage)	All good chemists.
Garlic Powder	Hofel's Pure Foods, Bury St. Edmunds, Suffolk.
Garlodex tablets	Healthcrafts Ltd.
Gelozone crystals (for jellies)	Modern Health Products. (Also most health-foods shops.)
Gestaal (Barley Germ)	F. E. Clarke Ltd., Seething Lane, London, E.C.3. (Health-foods shops will obtain.)
Gluten-free flour	Energen Co.
Hepata (for hepatitis)	Inter-Medics Ltd.
Herb teas	Potter's Herbal Supplies.

Remedial Product	*Supplied by*
Herbamare Vegetable Salt	Swiss Health Products, 209 Blackburn Road, Wheelton, Chorley, Lancs.
Hyperisan	Swiss Health Products.
Innerfresh herbs (laxative)	Healthcrafts Ltd.
Iceland Moss	Potter's Herbal Supplies.
Juices of plants and raw vegetables (powdered)	Hofel's Pure Foods Ltd.
Juices of raw vegetables (liquid form)	Most health-foods shops.
Linseed	Potter's Herbal Supplies.
Linomel (Linseed and honey cereal)	Rayner and Pennycook Ltd.
Liquifruta	Any good chemist.
Liver tablets	Organic Vitamin Co.
Lecithin tablets	Organic Vitamin Co.
Lacto-flora tablets	Organic Vitamin Co.
Natex preparations	Modern Health Products.
Nettles (powdered)	Hofel's Pure Foods Ltd.
Nutramin A	Dr. Gilbert's Health Foods, Grantham, Lincs.
Olbas Oil (for external use)	G. Ashley & Co., 104 Christchurch Road, London, S.W.2.
Papain compound tablets	Potter's Herbal Supplies.
Passigen tablets (insomnia)	Carter's Herbal Supplies, Shipley, Yorks.
Pro-vitamin A	Most health-foods shops.
Rose-hip tablets	Most health-foods shops.
Rhubarb-root powder	Any good chemist.
Rauwolfia tablets	Swiss Health Products, 209 Blackburn Road, Wheelton, Chorley, Lancs.
Rumex Ointment	Any homoeopathic chemist.
Rutin tea	Most health-foods shops.
Salus bath-salts	Rayner & Pennycook Ltd.

Remedial Product	*Supplied by*
Salus tea	Rayner & Pennycook Ltd.
Sauerkraut	Health-foods shops.
Slippery-elm food- beverage	Most health-foods shops.
Tromacaps (for cystitis)	Inter-Medics Ltd.
Urgenin (for prostatitis)	Inter-Medics Ltd.
Vegetex (for rheumatism)	Modern Health Products.
Vitamin B.12 (with intrinsic factor)	Health-foods shops.
Vitamin C (powder)	Health-foods shops.
Vinca Rosea herb	Potter's Herbal Supplies.
Dr. Gilbert's Biochemic Remedies	The Biochemic Centre, Gran- tham, Lincs.
Dr. Vogel remedies	Swiss Health Products.
Whey powder	British Biochemic Co., Gran- tham, Lincs.
Watercress (powdered)	Hofel's Pure Foods Ltd.
Yestamin (brewer's yeast powder)	Most health-foods shops.
Yoghourt	Most health-foods shops.

HERBAL RECIPES

Bean-pod soup. Chop up some runner-beans, and, after soaking them overnight, simmer them gently in this water, for 30–40 minutes. Then strain. Take ½ teacupful 3–4 times a day, between meals. Its value and flavour is enhanced by the addition of a sprinkling of garlic powder.

It is a valuable remedy for diabetes, rheumatism, kidney troubles, dropsy, gout, and heart weakness.

Comfrey tea. This can be made with either fresh or dried leaves, using 1 oz. of the leaves to 1 pint of boiling water. Simmer for 10 minutes, allow to stand (covered) till cold, then strain. Take frequent sips of it for all chest complaints;

also for all gastro-intestinal inflammations. Dust comfrey powder on varicose ulcers.

Camomile tea. This is made of dried flowers, exactly like Comfrey tea. It is taken for debility, depression, exhaustion, sleeplessness, failing appetite, indigestion, and for all nerve troubles.

Elderflower tea. This is a valuable remedy for use in fevers, feverish colds, appendicitis, and whenever sweating needs to be encouraged. It is made as follows:

Put $\frac{1}{2}$ oz. boneset, $\frac{1}{2}$ oz. cinnamon, and $\frac{1}{2}$ oz. elderflowers (fresh or dried) into an enamel saucepan. Cover with $1\frac{1}{2}$ pints of water. Bring slowly to the boil and allow to simmer for 30 minutes. (Keep the pan covered with a lid.) Strain into a jug. In another pan simmer (but do not bring to the boil) about $\frac{1}{2}$ oz. peppermint (fresh or dried) in $\frac{1}{2}$ pint of water, for 30 minutes. Strain into the same jug as the elderflower water. When cool add 1 teaspoonful of composition powder and a little honey to sweeten. Warm up the mixture and take frequent drinks of it, to promote sweating.

Linseed tea. Put 1 tablespoonful linseed and $\frac{1}{2}$ oz. stick liquorice-root into 2 pints of water in a saucepan; simmer gently for about 1 hour, then strain, add 1 tablespoonful of honey and the juice of $\frac{1}{2}$ lemon. Wonderful for coughs and colds; also constipation.

Nettle tea. Using about 2 oz. of nettles to 1 pint of water, this is made in exactly the same way as other herb-teas, except that, if fresh nettles are used, the water should be very hot but not boiling. The nettles should be steeped in it (in a covered saucepan) for $\frac{1}{2}$ hour, over a tiny flame of gas – just sufficient to keep up the temperature of the water but not to boil it. If dried nettles are used, they should be brought up to boil and simmered for $\frac{1}{2}$ hour. Nettle tea is a powerful blood-cleanser and nerve-strengthener, and should be taken frequently by people who suffer with rheumatism, gout, sciatica, neuritis, nettle-rash, shingles, blood-impurity, etc.

Parsley tea. This is made like other herb teas, using about 1 oz. fresh parsley (2 oz. dried) to 1 pint of water. It should be taken in teaspoonful doses, 3 or 4 times a day, by people who suffer with bladder troubles, kidney stone, gravel, dropsy, and gout.

SOME GOLDEN RULES OF HEALTH

Wherever there is garbage, Nature gets to work on it. Her workers are tiny microscopic creatures called bacteria. There are many kinds of bacteria, some beneficial to Man, some harmful. The beneficial kind give rise to fermentation, the harmful kind to putrefaction (a going-rotten process).

The normal inhabitants of the large bowel in Man – the bacilli Coli Communis, and the bacilli Acidophillus – are acid-forming beneficial bacteria, which break down the body's waste-products by a process of fermentation. This they can do only if the food-residues in the bowel contain 'roughage', i.e. carbohydrate wastes, such as the peel of vegetables and fruits, and the bran of grain. The lactic acid formed in the process of fermentation prevents the formation of putrefactive poisons and also acts as a stimulant to the bowel, encouraging normal evacuation.

But if the food-residues in the bowel contain no such cellulose material (roughage), the bacteria, feeding only on the incompletely digested portions of flesh foods, turn from friends into enemies – they become putrefactive, poison-producing organisms. Moreover, the growth of other kinds of harmful bacteria is encouraged by such surroundings. The result is foul-smelling products, atrophy of the bowel, constipation, and a vitamin and mineral starvation, owing to the fact that vitamins and minerals are found chiefly in the peel of fruits and vegetables, in the husks of grain, and in the green leaves and stems of vegetables. The overall result is that the beneficial bacteria gradually disappear altogether, being replaced by putrefactive poisons. Very often, the entire population of the large bowel of someone who eats flesh-foods consists of putrefactive poison-producing bacteria, and, as a consequence, his stools are foul-smelling.

Some roughage should, therefore, be eaten every day if the large bowel (the main drain of the body) is to be kept healthy and free from putrefactive poisons, which produce auto-intoxication, and foul-smelling stools. *This is Golden Rule number one.*

Every mouthful of food (and this includes milk) should be thoroughly chewed. Moreover, solid food should not be washed down with liquid of any kind, all liquids being taken between meals, never *with* them; also, over-hot and ice-cold foods (and drinks) should be avoided. *This is Golden Rule number two.*

The body should be washed all over every day and frictioned with a brush or rough towel. No soap should be used, except for the removal of dirt from the hands or other exposed parts of the body, but a rub all over with common salt followed by a cool shower is very beneficial. The temperature of the water should not exceed 98.4°F. Hot baths (except on occasion for some special purpose such as to induce sweating) are relaxing and weakening. *Skin hygiene* is, therefore, *Golden Rule number three.*

The rooms in which you live, eat, and sleep should be well-ventilated, so that at all times of the day and night you are breathing pure oxygen-rich air. *This is Golden Rule number four.*

Daily exercise (preferably the sort that induces sweating, because by means of sweating the body is able to eliminate waste-products and toxins) is *Golden Rule number five*. Without exercise, the body is unable to manufacture its own digestive enzymes. Exercise also stimulates the circulation of the blood and ensures that it is properly oxygenated. If for any reason you are unable to take exercise, you should step-up your intake of *raw* foods, as those are the only sort that contain enzymes; cooking destroys vitamins and enzymes in food. (The other reason why food should be eaten in its natural raw state, as far as possible, is because it provides better roughage.)

Golden Rule number six is 'Eat only when hungry'. Remember that, because first-class protein food contains *all* the essential amino-acids, it is not necessary nor advisable to eat more than one first-class protein at any meal. This does not mean that two different kinds of cheese or two different kinds of fish should not be eaten at the same meal; it simply means that two or three different kinds of first-class protein should not be eaten together; for example, meat and fish are different kinds of first-class protein; so are meat and poultry; so are meat and milk, and it simply overburdens the digestive organs if these combinations are eaten together.

It is not generally realized that thousands more people die of over-eating than of starvation. Democritus, the Greek scientist who lived to be 109, advocated a sparse diet as the recipe for a long life. So, never eat to repletion – always get up from the table feeling that you could, if necessary, eat a little more – and never be persuaded to eat when you feel no desire for food, nor when you are over-tired or exhausted, or emotionally upset, or in a bad mood. Food at such times will not be properly digested; it is better not to eat till the tiredness or the upset or the mood has passed, or till you feel a real desire for food.

Golden Rule number seven is 'Never eat what you positively dislike, but try to like the right things'. The right things are the natural whole unrefined foods, fresh-picked vegetables, salads, fruits, etc., eaten, as far as possible, in their raw state. (Raw vegetables can be juiced in a juice-press.)

Soft mushy foods, like porridge and packet cereals soaked in milk, should be replaced by raw bran and raw oatmeal or groats (ground oat-grains). These should be soaked for 10–15 minutes in a little boiling water before eating them; then milk and a little honey may be added. Refined white sugar should be avoided; so, too, should flesh foods, which, to make palatable, need cooking, and cooking kills their vitamins and digestive-enzymes, without which they cannot be completely digested and assimilated by the human digestive organs. This leads inevitably to auto-intoxication (self-poisoning) and disease. Eskimos are big meat-eaters, yet they are very disease-free, cancer being unknown amongst them. This is due to the fact that they eat their meat raw, thereby conserving its digestive enzymes, thus enabling it to be completely digested and assimilated by the digestive organs.

Golden Rule number eight is 'Take a short rest before and after meals'. Rest, if possible, in the body-slant position, i.e. with your feet and legs higher than your heart. A special chair for relaxation (it is called a relaxator) can be bought. Resting in the body-slant position promotes a better circulation and relieves the work of the heart, by reversing the pull of gravity on the blood-flow. It also relieves congestion in the legs and feet, assists the digestive organs, and helps to relax all muscles and nerves.

Golden Rule number nine is 'Give your digestive organs an occasional rest by going without solid food for 24 hours – say, from after breakfast one morning till the same time next day'. During that time, some liquid can and should be taken, drinks of herb-tea, diluted fruit-juices, and vegetable juices are best.

Golden Rule number ten is 'Start every meal with something raw'. This prevents leucocytosis (a flooding of the digestive tract with leucocytes). Leucocytes are the white blood-cells which form the defence-corps of the body; they are called upon to defend the body against invading foreign substances, diseases, germs, etc. For millions of years Man lived on raw unfired foods, and has not yet entirely 'adapted' to cooked foods. These are, therefore, still foreign to his alimentary tract, and, every time they are eaten, they cause a calling-up of the defence-corps. This constant calling-up of the militia weakens the defence-mechanism of the body. To avoid it, all that is necessary is to eat something raw before you eat your cooked food; this cancels the alarm signal (so to speak), and the militia is not called upon to defend the body against the 'foreign' (cooked) food that follows the raw food.

COMPATIBLE AND INCOMPATIBLE FOODS

To combine foods correctly is as essential and important a pre-requisite of good health as to choose them correctly. It does not involve omitting any of the chosen ones – it simply means getting into the habit of eating the incompatible ones at different meal-times. In other words, we can continue to eat exactly the same foods (provided that they are natural whole foods), but we should combine them in such a way that incompatible ones are not eaten together at the same meal. For example, protein foods (meat, poultry, fish, cheese, eggs, etc.) need acid juices in the stomach for their digestion, and, for the most part, they should not be eaten together with carbonaceous foods (starchy foods), because they need an alkaline medium for their digestion. If they *are* eaten together, the flow of acid juices in the stomach is inhibited, and the digestion of both the protein *and* the carbohydrate foods is adversely affected and seriously slowed up. However, as explained on page 22, a portion of one's daily intake of protein-food *should* be eaten with a slice of bread (or some other form of carbohydrate food) to ensure that it is used for body-building purposes.

Fruit of all kinds (acid, semi-sweet, and sweet) has the same inhibiting effect on the flow of gastric acids when eaten with protein foods, and should not, therefore, be eaten with them. Neither should acid or semi-sweet fruit be eaten with starchy foods, because the acid of the fruit destroys the alkalinity of the saliva which initiates the digestion of starchy foods. In fact, acid fruit retards the digestion of all food with which it is eaten (except perhaps nuts), so it should be eaten by itself – one sort at a time.

Sweet fruits (such as dates, figs, sultanas, raisins, and bananas), contain no free acid, so they may be eaten with starchy foods, but, actually, *all* kinds of fruit are best eaten by themselves – not with other foods. They make an ideal breakfast. The three kinds of fruit (acid, semi-sweet, and sweet), should not, of course, be mixed and eaten together at the same time; neither should fruit be eaten *between* meals.

Acid fruits include oranges, lemons, grapefruits, gooseberries, plums, red and black currants. Semi-sweet fruits include dessert apples, pears, grapes, melons, avocados, peaches, apricots, cherries, greengages, etc. Sweet fruits include dates, figs, bananas, sultanas and raisins. Avocados contain some protein. (See *Food-combining made easy*, by Dr. Tilden. Also *Superior Nutrition*, by Dr. Shelton.)

Correct food-combining and the separation of incompatible foods play an all-important part in the body's ability to recover from illness. The explanation for this is as follows:

The digestion of protein foods takes place in seven stages. If it is slowed up as a result of the protein having been eaten together with starch, sugar, or fats, the protein gets absorbed into the bloodstream at the fourth stage, the peptone stage, before it has reached the amino-acid stage, the fully-digested stage. This results in a clogging of the intercellular spaces with semi-digested protein-products at the peptone stage of digestion, and this impedes not only the free circulation of the intercellular fluids carrying the body-nutrients, the all-important mineral salts, and oxygen to the cells, but the collection of waste-products *from* the cells. The consequence of such impeding is cell-deterioration, and a diminution of nervous energy, and of the body's powers of recuperation from illness. These can be built up only by freeing the inter-cellular fluids of semi-digested protein waste-products (peptones) so that they can flow freely round the cells and nourish them properly.

Protein foods (animal and vegetable) are more easily and quickly digested if eaten with green leafy vegetables (or salad crops), cooked or raw. The protein meal should contain no starch or sugar foods (other than one slice of bread or one medium-size potato), no animal fats, and no fruit, as these all retard its digestion and promote its absorption into the bloodstream at the semi-digested (peptone) stage. The only stage at which it can be completely assimilated by the body, after its absorption, is the seventh stage, the amino-acid stage.

The digestion of fats is a long and complicated process. There is a fat-splitting enzyme in the gastric juice, but the chief part of fat-digestion takes place in the small intestine where the fats are emulsified (softened) by bile-juice and then split into fatty-acids and glycerol by pancreatic enzymes. Fat-digestion (fat-oxidation) can be carried to a successful conclusion only if carbohydrates are present. If fat is eaten without some starchy food, its digestion stops short at the aceto-acetic acid stage; the acid gets converted into other toxic substances, and accumulates in the body.

Two meals a day, plus a fruit breakfast, should suffice most people. One of the meals should be an all-protein meal, consisting of one 'complete' protein food (a food that contains *all* the essential amino-acids) and one or two 'incomplete' ones. If the meal consists only of several 'incomplete' protein foods (i.e. foods in which one or more of the essential amino-acids are missing, such as nuts, grains, seeds, pulses, or soya-beans) they should be selected so that their amino-acids complement each other, together forming a 'complete' protein. (See 'How to be Healthy on a Vegetarian or Vegan Diet' page 229.)

The protein meal can include potatoes and green vegetables and/or salads, but no fruit, and no animal fats. The other meal should be a chiefly carbonaceous one, i.e. one that excludes acid fruits, but includes potatoes, green vegetables, egg, salad dressed with vegetable oil, wholewheat bread or toast, a little unsalted butter, and about 2 oz. of cottage or St. Ivel cream cheese. It can include banana, sweet dried fruits, such as dates, figs, or raisins. Plantmilk can be taken with the fruit.

Raw milk is an almost complete food. Its protein content is 56% and it contains calcium and other important mineral salts, also vitamin A if it comes from cows fed on lush meadow grass and carrots. It is best taken with bread or cereals, being rich in fats. If taken by itself, it should be diluted with a little water or soda-water to make it more digestible, and only in small quantities.

The eating of flesh food is not advised. Cooking destroys its digestive enzymes, without which it cannot be completely digested; the result is a clogging of the body's intercellular spaces with semi-digested proteins (peptones), and consequent interference with cell-respiration and cell-nutrition. This is inevitably followed by cell-deterioration, a lowering of cell-resistance, and a diminution of nervous energy.

MENTAL HEALTH

Most physical ills are caused by bad physical habits; likewise many mental ills are caused by bad mental habits.

A habit is the repetition of something that started as only a tendency, but the tendency wore a groove, and then became a habit. People who have the responsibility of rearing children should remember this and try to get them to establish good habits early in life when the mind is virgin and ungrooved, like a blank record-disc. Once the grooves have made their impression on the disc, with each repeat they grow more difficult to smooth out and eradicate. A long-standing habit is powerful and therefore very difficult to break.

Eating habits can become bad, like the habit of smoking or swearing. But all bad habits can be broken. It is best to tackle them one at a time, *not* all at once, and the time to start is now – not tomorrow or next week.

Each conquest of a bad habit strengthens the will. To do anything worthwhile requires will-power, and will-power will grow in strength through exercising it, just as muscles become stronger the more they are exercised. Conquering bad physical habits helps us to conquer harmful negative emotions, such as anger, fear, worry, hatred, jealousy, envy, spite, self-pity, etc., all of which are bad for our physical health.

So, just as bad physical habits can be conquered by will-power, so too can bad mental and emotional habits. Exercise of the will turns wish-power into will-power, just as walking exercise turns weak leg muscles into strong ones.

All negative emotions poison the blood, and, as anger is the most violent of these emotions, it produces the worst form of poisoning; it produces tension of the whole body, which saps one's nervous energy, and this causes enervation and consequent toxaemia.

The best way to conquer anger, therefore, is to relax all your muscles – muscles of the face, of the head and neck, of the arms and hands, of the whole body. This physical relaxation will relax mental and emotional tension, and your anger will fade.

Fear, also, breeds a poison in the body and causes food to remain undigested in the stomach; so, too, does worry, which is really a form of fear – a less powerful but equally harmful form. Worry destroys the power to think clearly; it causes indigestion with flatulence and acidity, and these cause heart pains and nervous irritability. Worrying can never prevent a thing happening, nor cure it if it *has* happened. It makes any bodily disease worse, and tends to retard recovery. It is a completely negative and useless emotion – and anyway 'Why worry, it may never happen', as the saying is.

Sometimes an under-active thyroid gland or a functionally disturbed one is the cause of mental disease. The disturbance of the gland can be caused by constant dosing with aspirin; or by over-indulgence in the use of stimulants (tea, coffee, and cigarette-smoking). The under-activity of the gland can be due to an iodine deficiency in the blood. This can be remedied by eating foods rich in iodine such as sea-foods, and by taking 3–4 kelp tablets a day. (Kelp is dried seaweed.)

A healthy thyroid gland, functioning normally is indispensable to mental health, mental activity, and freedom from depression. The hormones it secretes control the rate at which the body oxidizes its food-supply; this means that the gland has an enormous effect upon blood-sugar level and thus upon the mental outlook of its owner, mental depression being the inevitable result of a low blood-sugar level.

The secretions from the thyroid are also essential for helping in the transportation of oxygen to the brain – mental disorders being very often due to an oxygen-deficiency in the brain.

The efficiency of the gland can be restored to normal by taking foods rich in vitamin B such as brewer's yeast, wheat-germ cereal, foods made of soya-beans such as 'Granogen' and 'Plantmilk'. Extra vitamin C is also required. This can be obtained from acerola or rose-hip tablets. It may also be necessary to take Thyroid extract, but your doctor will order this if he thinks it necessary.

All endocrine glands are directly influenced by morbid thoughts and feelings – as also by their converse. The nature of one's emotions can thus restrict or release essential hormones that maintain the delicate balance of health. The endocrine glands are the first to respond to mental or emotional changes. For example, when terribly depressed, the slowed-down release of hormones (chemical messengers) from the endocrine glands induces a heightened degree of susceptibility to disease-elements. Conversely, when happy and elated, there is a heightened release of hormones from the glands and a consequent strengthening of resistance to encroaching disease-elements.

We read 'It is certain that your sins will find you out'. By 'sins' is meant negative mental and emotional states, such as anger, envy, jealousy, worry, frustration, depression, and fear.

Thus it can be truly said that, to a great extent, we can control our own health – or lack of health.

DR. BACH'S FLOWER REMEDIES

The remedies used in this method of healing are all prepared from the flowers of wild plants, bushes, and trees, and none of them are harmful or habit-forming.

They are prescribed not for the sufferer's physical complaint but for his worry, fear, depression, or irritability, because these states of mind not only hinder recovery of health and retard convalescence but are the primary causes of sickness and disease.

A long-continued worry or fear, as is well known, will deplete the individual's vitality; he will feel out of sorts, below par, not himself. His body then loses its natural resistance to disease and is in a fit state to become the prey of any infection and of any form of illness, whether it be the common cold, rheumatism, digestive disturbance, or more serious diseases. So it is the patient himself – the sufferer from the complaint – who needs treatment, *not* the complaint. As peace and harmony return to his mind, health will also return to his body.

This method of treatment, and the remedies, were discovered by a doctor who had practised for over twenty years in London as a Harley Street consultant, bacteriologist, and homoeopath. The late Edward Bach, M.B., B.S., M.R.C.S., L.R.C.P., D.P.H., gave up his lucrative practice in 1930 to devote his time to research work on these lines, and to seek the plant remedies which would restore vitality to the sick, so that the sufferer himself would be able to overcome his worry, his fear, or his depression, and so effect his own healing.

There are thirty-eight Bach remedies, one for each of the thirty-eight negative states of mind (or moods) common to mankind. These states of mind are divided into seven groups under the following headings: fear; uncertainty; insufficient interest in present circumstances; loneliness; over-sensitivity to influences and ideas; despondency or despair; and over-care for the welfare of others.

Under the heading of fear, for instance, are five remedies for the five different kinds of fear. These are classified as terror, fear of known cause, fear of *un*known cause, fear of the mind losing control, and fear for other people.

The remedy for terror (or extreme fear) is given when the patient, or those around him, are feeling great fear because the illness is so severe and there is little hope of his or her recovery; it is also given for the fear felt in acute illness or accidents. The nature or name of the illness makes no difference – if terror is present, then the remedy for terror is the one the patient requires.

There is a remedy for the after-effects of shock, whether it be mental or physical in origin. There is one for impatience, for extreme tension and irritability of mind which results in tension and pain in the body. There is another for drowsiness, faintness, or unconsciousness; this remedy comes under the heading 'lack of interest in present circumstances'. There is also a remedy for that state of despair when the sufferer feels that he may lose control and feels the impulse to do dreaded and unwished-for things. These last five remedies are also combined to form one remedy called the Rescue remedy. This is a first-aid remedy, invaluable in times of emergency, accident, shock, and sudden illness, for it can be given to

211

soothe and calm the patient until other measures can be taken.

It will be seen that these five remedies meet all emergency states – terror, shock, unconsciousness, tension, pain, and loss of control.

As the Bach flower remedies are benign in their action and can result in no unpleasant reactions, they can be used by anyone. They can also be taken at the same time as any other medicine or treatment, if so desired, without affecting the result of either.

All that need be remembered is 'Treat the patient and *not* the disease'. Treat the fear, the indecision, the depondency or hopelessness of the patient, no matter what the name of his illness is.

If desired, treatment can be obtained from members of Dr. Bach's team. Patients can be seen by appointment at headquarters in Wallingford, Berks. (the address is The Bach Healing Centre, Mount Vernon, Sotwell, Wallingford, Berks.). Advice and remedies are also available by post.

If the patient wishes to treat himself, a price-list of stock bottles of the thirty-eight remedies can be obtained from the Secretary at the Healing Centre.

The six books (all published by The C. W. Daniel Co. Ltd., 60 Muswell Road, London, N.10) recommended for reading in connection with flower-healing work are:

Handbook of the Bach Flower Remedies by Philip Chancellor.
The Twelve Healers by Edward Bach.
Heal Thyself by Edward Bach.
The Bach Remedies Repertory by F. J. Wheeler.
The Medical Discoveries of Edward Bach by Nora Weeks.
The Bach Flower Remedies by Nora Weeks and Victor Bullen.

There is also a quarterly publication, the *Bach Remedy Newsletter*, available from the Bach Healing Centre.

RADIESTHESIA

Radiesthesia is akin to dowsing, which is the practice of detecting and locating the presence of underground water. Dowsing is practised by people sensitive to, and able to pick up, the radiations (energy-waves) given off by water. Radiesthesia (sometimes called 'psionic medicine') is medical dowsing.

Everything in Nature radiates energy-waves (inorganic as well as organic substances) and these waves can be picked up by a sensitive piece of apparatus, just as sound waves can be picked up by a microphone. All living creatures radiate energy-waves, and these can be picked up, and measured, by radiesthesia apparatus.

Our ancestors would have scoffed at the idea of radio, television and telephones, and would have thought them impossible, for, as is well known, nearly all great inventions are at first thought impossible and their creators ignored or ridiculed. But, to those who understand electricity or electronics, the apparatus that measures human radiations is no more mysterious than the radio, television, telephone, or geiger-counter. Apparently, the tuning-means of radiesthesia apparatus are based upon radio-engineering practices, which use inductance and capacity in the same manner as for the tuning-in of radio sets. The delicate radio-like radiesthesia instrument picks up the electrical signals from each organ or tissue of the patient's body (each of which has its own characteristic wavelength, i.e. its own radio-signal). These signals, according to their strength or weakness, indicate the strength or weakness of the 'vital force' in the organ or tissue. Thus, by turning dials, the operator, like a radio-operator picking up various stations, can detect the strong or weak signals from the various organs or tissues, and, by comparing them with the frequency-rates (previously tested) of healthy and diseased organs and tissues, can determine the condition of each organ or tissue of the patient. If a patient is unable to go to a radiesthesia practitioner, a sample of blood or sputum can be sent instead, and the practitioner can diagnose this (by means of the energy-waves it radiates) equally successfully.

Thus, by means of radiesthesia, it seems to be possible to diagnose not only established disease in an organ or tissue, but 'disease-tendencies'; also to *locate* these tendencies, long before any outward signs or symptoms are detected by the patient himself or by his doctor.

This, surely, is PREVENTIVE MEDICINE par excellence.

For further reading on the subject, see the following:

Get Well Naturally (Chapter 12) by Linda Clark (Devin-Adair Co., New York).

An Introduction to Radiesthesia by Dr. Vernon Wethered (C. W. Daniel).

The Pattern of Health by Dr. Westlake (Davin-Adair Co.).

Principles and Practices of Radiesthesia by Abbé Mermet (T. Nelson & Co., New York).

New Light on Therapeutic Energies by Mark Gallert (James Clark & Co., London).

A CANCER THERAPY

According to Dr. Howard Beard, author of *A New Approach to the Conquest of Cancer*, human malignancy is, biochemically speaking, a chymotrypsin (and a nutritional) 'deficiency' disease.

Chymotrypsin is an enzyme produced by the pancreas. If there is an over-abundance of anti-chymotrypsin (which is also self-produced), a malignant growth will result.

About 80% of people are able to produce sufficient pancreatic chymotrypsin to prevent them from ever developing cancer; the other 20% are not able to produce sufficient, and tumours will develop (benign or malignant, according to the pre-natal nature of their component cells) *unless preventive steps are taken*. These steps are:

A preliminary testing of the urine for the presence in it of chorionic gonadatrophin (hormones produced by trophoblastic (malignant) tissue-cells). This is called the Anthrone Test. It will reveal a developing tumour years before it shows up clinically.

If the result of the test is positive, injections of chymotrypsin (pancreatic enzymes) and of Laetrile (a synthetic drug containing benzaldehyde, glucuronic acid, and hydrocyanic acid) should be begun immediately, even though no signs or symptoms of a growth have shown themselves. These steps will *prevent* the formation of a growth, and prevention is the only sure cure; although, even if it has started to grow, it is curable if it is treated by chemotherapy (as above) before any clinical signs of its existence show themselves.

The test should be carried out every six months after the age of 40, every 3 months after the age of 60, and every 2 months after the age of 70. Only thus can cancer be caught in the early stages of its growth and treated successfully. Treatment would not, of course, be necessary if the result of the test were negative, but, if it were positive (i.e. if the urine were found to contain chorionic gonadatrophin), injections of chymotrypsin should be given, and repeated at regular intervals until the result of testing becomes negative, and remains negative.

Synthetic galactose laetrile is injected into a vein, and reaches the tumour via the blood, where it meets with the blood-enzyme beta-glucuronidase. The result is an immediate triggering of HCN (hydrocyanic acid); this stops all tumour-respiration, and death of the tumour-cells is the result. The fact that the normal cells are not also killed is due to the presence in them of the enzyme rhodanese; this inactivates the HCN as soon as it is liberated.

Pregnancy and malignancy closely resemble each other – indeed, they are analogous processes. The former is a natural physiological process; the latter is, from the clinical point of view, unnatural and pathological.

It seems strangely incongruous of Nature to have provided trophoblastic (malignant) cell-tissue in pregnancy (for the maintenance and welfare of the placenta), whose behaviour in any other location of the body (i.e. outside of pregnancy) would be tumour-forming. It is extremely fortunate that Nature has also provided each one of us with chymotrypsin (pancreatic enzyme) to hold the trophoblastic tissue in check; if this were not the case, all living creatures (including man) would be born with a beginning cancer.

Sometimes, when a woman with cancer becomes pregnant, a spontaneous recovery takes place. Dr. Beard says this can only be explained by the fact that, as soon as the pancreas of the foetus begins to develop at 7 weeks after conception, the chymotrypsin it produces is added to the chymotrypsin produced by the mother's pancreas (insufficient in itself), and the combined amounts are sufficient to destroy the trophoblastic (malignant) tissue in her body.

The placental trophoblastin also begins to disappear at about this time (it is destroyed by the chymotrypsin produced by the developing foetal pancreas), having served its purpose in providing for the growth of the placenta, the nutrition of the embryo, and the elimination of waste-products from the foetus. Its disappearance is coincident with, and proved by, the excretion in the mother's urine of chorionic gonadatrophin (hormones produced by tropho-blastic cells). The excretion of these hormones, at this time, is the highest of the whole pregnancy; it steadily decreases thenceforth to almost none at all.

Dr. Beard says that a malignant tumour should never be removed surgically, though surgery to remove the somatic remains of it, *after treatment with Laetrile and with chymo-trypsin*, may be advisable.

Another substance that is also injected for a malignant tumour is Pangamic acid (vitamin B.15). Trophoblastic (malignant) cells, of which the tumour is formed, thrive in an atmosphere of carbon-dioxide, but will die in the presence of oxygen. Since one of the important functions of this vitamin is to increase the supply and utilization of oxygen in the tissues, we can see that it will produce an unfavourable environment for the propagation of cancer-cells and tissues. We can see that it must also be a substance that is of great importance in the treatment of all heart troubles, because the great need in heart troubles is for oxygen.

Pangamic acid (vitamin B.15) can be regarded as a pre-ventive measure as well as a curative one. It seems to be unobtainable in England, but is obtainable in America. An address from which to obtain it is: House of Nutrition, 1125, 6th Avenue, San Diego, California, U.S.A.

In the writer's opinion everyone over the age of 40 should take it (or vitamin E which is a good substitute for it) every day.

With the passing of the years, i.e. as we get older, the hormonal balance between the pancreas and the Adrenal glands becomes upset, the pancreas producing less and less insulin (possibly less and less chymotrypsin too), and the Adrenals producing no less adrenalin; this causes a surplus of adrenalin in the blood, one effect of which is an increase of tension throughout the body. (There may be other effects about which we know nothing at present.)

It is thought by Professor Nikitin (Biochemist) of Krakov University, that hormonal balance can be restored by be-coming hungry, through fasting for short periods, now and then. Hunger causes the semi-digested protein foods we eat, which clog the intercellular spaces, to be seized by the blood when it becomes desperate for nourishment (as it does when we fast) and thus to be digested and then excreted from the body; for it is clogging of the intercellular spaces, *as well as an over-abundance of adrenalin in the blood*, that causes degenerative diseases, because clogging of these spaces means that oxygen cannot reach the cells, their respiration is thus interfered with, and their metabolism disturbed. This sets the scene for the development of cell-deterioration and consequent disease. So a day or two, now and then, without solid food is advisable.

Insulin treatment for cancer. This lowers the blood-sugar level, thus setting free more oxygen for cell-nourishment. It should be given in addition to Pangamic acid (vitamin B.15), which, as already explained, increases the supply and utilization of oxygen in the tissues, thus producing an unfavourable atmosphere for the propagation of cancer-cells and tissues, which die in the presence of oxygen.

HOMOEOPATHY

Homoeopathic healing is based on the principle that 'like cures like'. This is in direct contrast to orthodox (allopathic) healing which is based on the principle that 'opposite cures opposite'.

What it means is that a patient is given a very minute dose of a substance that, if given to normal healthy people in large doses, would produce the symptoms of the patient's illness. It is a system of healing that was first recorded by the Greek physician Hippocrates in the fifth century B.C., then by the physician Paracelsus in the seventeenth century, being perfected by Hahnemann in the nineteenth century.

The medicinal substances used in homoeopathic medicines can be of animal, vegetable, or mineral origin. Such a substance is made into a medicine as follows: It is first ground into a fine powder; then one part of this powder is mixed with nine parts of milk-sugar and the two substances are pounded together for several hours. The resulting medicine is what is termed a 1x. preparation, and it contains only one tenth of the original medicinal substance. A preparation of a higher 'potency' is made by mixing together one part of the 1x. preparation and another nine parts of milk-sugar. This mixture is likewise pounded for several hours, and the result is a 2x. preparation, which contains only one hundredth part of the original substance. Such a dilution process (it is called 'trituration') can be repeated and repeated, the result of each repeat being a diminution in the amount of the original substance in the resulting preparation. For example, a third repeat results in a 3x. preparation which contains only a thousandth part of the original substance (the substance that, if given in large doses to healthy people, produces the symptoms of the patient's illness). A 6x. preparation contains only a millionth part, and a 12x. only a trillionth part.

It will be realized therefore that the amount of actual substance remaining in a preparation of a 6x. (or higher) potency is negligible. Yet homoeopathic doctors say that the higher the potency, the greater is the effect on the body of the sick person, the very high potencies producing the most pronounced physical reactions. Such a statement is disputed by allopathic doctors who are unable to accept and believe that such a medicine, which contains less than one molecule of the original substance, has any effect on the body at all. However, homoeopathic medicines *do* seem to produce physical reactions, not only in the human body but in the bodies of animals (veterinary surgeons who use them will vouch for this), so the idea that the reaction in a human body might be due to wishful thinking or to auto-suggestion can, it would seem, be discarded.

The dilution of liquid substances is done by vigorously shaking together 1 drop of the crude substance with 99 drops of spirit of alcohol. The resulting medicine is a 'first potency' preparation and has the figure 1 after its name, e.g. Calendula 1. To produce a preparation of the 2nd potency, 1 drop of this Calendula 1 preparation is shaken up ('succussed') with another 99 drops of spirit of alcohol. The process of dilution can be continued for up to 100 times, sometimes more.

The medicinal substances used in the making of homoeopathic medicine are tried out ('proved') on healthy volunteers. Each 'prover' is asked to note any changes from normal health caused by taking the substance (it is taken in large allopathic doses), and to report such changes to the doctor who is conducting the 'proving'. Each substance is 'proved' by a group of people (men, women, and children) of different ages and types. These people do not know what they are taking, and they do not see or talk to each other. The 'proving' may last for several weeks, at the end of which time the doctor arranges the resulting symptoms according to the part of the 'prover's' body to have been affected, e.g. the head, the sense-organs, the abdomen, the back, the chest, the limbs, etc. The symptoms are arranged also according to how the 'prover's' sleep, dreams, nerves, or personality have been affected.

About 500 substances have been 'proved', and their sum-total is the 'materia-medica' of homoeopathic prescribing. In addition, there are about 1,500 other substances that have been proved, but which are used only rarely.

Sick people, whose symptoms of ill-health correspond with the symptoms produced in the 'provers' by the taking of the crude substance, are given doses of the substance in homoeopathic form (i.e. triturated) in a potency varying from 1x. to 30x. (or higher), according to their sensitivity and temperament, according also to the length of time they have had the symptoms of ill-health. Generally speaking, long-standing (chronic) symptoms are treated with higher potency remedies, acute symptoms (short-term ones) with lower potency remedies. For very long-standing symptoms, the potency can be as high as 200, but such a high potency dose is usually given only once, or at most twice with a long interval between the two doses.

The fact that the same remedy can be (and is) given in different potencies (low, medium, or high, according to the sensitivity of the patient and to the length of time he has had the symptoms of illness) makes homoeopathic healing unique. It also makes it more difficult to practise successfully.

The homoeopathic doctor has not only to choose the right remedy (to match the totality of the symptoms), in the right potency (to match the patient's sensitivity), but he has also to take into consideration the patient's environment and inherited disease-tendencies ('miasms'). These tendencies can block the free flow of vital energy, and must be removed before he can hope to cure the patient's illness. They are usually the result of suppression of symptoms (in the patient's parents) by suppressive drugs which have driven the symptoms inwards, and these symptoms emerge, maybe many years later, in the children of the parents. The homoeopathic doctor, to remove any such inherited disease-tendency, gives first the remedy which the parent should have been given instead of the drug he (or she) *was* given. It is usually given in a very high potency, and one dose is usually sufficient, though it may take some time to produce any effect. Remedies to remove inherited disease-tendencies are called 'nosodes'.

It will be realized that homoeopathic prescribing is therefore a very difficult and complex art. It is fraught with almost insuperable difficulties and factors that have to be taken into consideration, and this means that a homoeopathic doctor's successes may be fewer than his failures.

Homoeopathic treatment is also a comparatively slow process, covering sometimes a period of many months. But 'slow is sure', as the saying is, and at least homoeopathic remedies have no harmful side-effects, as do allopathic drugs; nor do they clog the body with drug-residues (as do allopathic drugs) which often have toxic effects and initiate chronic degenerative diseases later in life. They are slower-acting than drugs, but much safer; moreover, they are selected to treat the individual, and to treat the whole of him (or her), not just his or her physical body.

HYDROTHERAPY

Hydrotherapy, the treatment of disease by water, was the basis of all healing in Greek and Roman times. The Roman baths at Bath, built by the Romans during their occupation of Britain, are still there and still being used, although the great aqueducts that conveyed the water to the baths are no longer used (the water was, of course, rainwater).

Hydrotherapy does not achieve as much nowadays as it did in those days, because the water now used is not rainwater, with its high sun-and-oxygen content and its innate powers of cleansing and of healing; also because it is not usually accompanied by fasting (or semi-fasting) or by diet-reform – at least, not in Gt. Britain. At the Bircher-Benner Clinic, near Zurich, it *is* accompanied by diet-reform, I believe, and is therefore more beneficial.

Hippocrates, the first real physician, who lived in Greece 2,400 years ago, was of the opinion that all disease is caused by a lack of oxygen in the blood and tissues. Oxygen, he said, is 'lord of all' – essential not only for human life and health, but also for animal and plant life, and even fire cannot live (i.e. burn) without it. He strongly advocated the use of rainwater which he called 'sunwater', both externally *and* internally, together with the raw juices of ripe fruits and vegetables. These, he said, by virtue of their oxygen-and-sunwater content, would provide the body with the necessary power to cast out its own disease, which it would do through the excretory organs, especially through the skin by means of boils or abscesses. These, he said, occur if disease *is* present in the body, and they should be helped to come to a head, and to discharge their toxins, by application of warm rainwater compresses, as also by daily bathing in warm rainwater or sea-water. The water treatment should be accompanied by much rest, fresh air, and sunlight, and by an adequate but sparse diet consisting mainly of fresh and ripe raw fruits and vegetables, and, if thirsty, sips of rainwater. (The digestion of food takes energy; therefore, because much energy is needed for self-cleansing and self-restorative purposes, the patient should not eat to repletion.)

Rainwater is full of the electro-dynamic energy of the sun, whose power draws it up from the earth into the clouds, from whence it descends as rain. Fruits, vegetables, and plants are nourished by the rainwater in the soil in which they are growing, so they, too, are full of 'sunwater'.

Rainwater contains not only solar energy and 30% more oxygen than tapwater, but also twice as much nitrogen, and nitrogen is essential for the building and repair of body-cells. Rainwater is also much lighter, purer, and less dense than tapwater (to which many chemicals are added nowadays). It has therefore the power to push and to penetrate into the minutest and remotest of the body-cells, and to supply them with oxygen, which is as vital to them as the food, the vitamins, and the minerals that they receive. Indeed, it is thought by some eminent authorities that one of the causes of cancer could be a lack of oxygen in the blood and lymph.

The profound effect that rainwater has upon the human body is clearly, simply, and convincingly explained in a wonderful book called *Healing by Water* by T. Hartley-Hennessy (The C. W. Daniel Co., 60 Muswell Road, London N.10). As the author says, one often hears the remark – 'So-and-So has frequent boils, and must therefore be very run-down.' Nothing could be further from the truth. Anyone who has sufficient vitality to cast out poisons from his body by means of boils must be in excellent health. Sick people who have insufficient vitality to produce such outlets are to be pitied, for, if they *had* such outlets, they would soon recover their health. Such vitality is a power quite different from, and beyond, the power of a doctor to heal. It is obtainable only from Nature – from fresh air rich in oxygen, from oxygenated sunwater (as found in ripe fruits and vegetables), from drinking (and bathing in) rainwater, and from natural whole foods grown in naturally-fertilized soils.

Faith and Hope and 'the will to live' are also powerful factors in the body's ability to summon up enough vitality to throw off disease – as also to resist it. No doctor can help someone who has no desire to live, and the most skilled surgeon can only 'set' a broken bone; it is Nature – one's own vitality – that knits the broken ends together and heals the tissues.

Ancient and modern medicine are in direct opposition to one another. Ancient science taught that all healing would come from the sunlight (solar energy) contained in living plants and fruits, and in rainwater, which would strengthen the recuperative powers of the body. Modern science teaches that healing can be effected by the use of man-made drugs. But these are foreign to the body (i.e. they are substances that do not enter into the composition of any of the body-cells); all that they do, therefore, is to give the body more work to do, because the body has to eject them as rapidly as possible, and they therefore hinder rather than help healing.

Modern science teaches that it is of no importance how dense our water is, how devoid of sunlight, oxygen, electrical forces and voltages from lightning, etc., or how polluted (by domestic and commercial wastes), so long as it is made safe for drinking by being chemically treated with chlorine, etc.

Modern science is also responsible for the fact that, in some parts of the country, water is being used (mis-used, really) as a vehicle for conveying sodium-fluoride to consumers – (a substance that is supposed to delay dental decay in children's teeth, but which has been proved to be not only valueless dentally, but harmful to many people). The practice of adding sodium-fluoride to water is tantamount to medicating it; moreover, it is enforced medication, since everyone in these fluoridated areas of the country is obliged to drink it (unless he goes to the expense and trouble of sinking a private well). Such a practice is unethical, and contrary to democratic principles.

From the moment that this 'doctored' water is replaced by sun-and-oxygen-rich rainwater, deterioration of body-tissues ceases and restoration begins. Bone-repair, for example, is a very slow process; bones grow at the same rate as plants, and it may be many months before complete healing takes place. This applies not only to damaged bones but also to other tissues and organs of the body; for healing is slow but sure.

In ancient times, hydropathy was used extensively by the Greek doctor Hippocrates (and others), who placed pads of soft linen soaked in rainwater over any painful or diseased part of a sick person's body, in the hope of producing a boil or small eruption, through which the causative poisons might be drained from the body.

Unfortunately, many sick people have such low vitality that even sun-and-oxygen-rich rainwater (used internally as well as externally) will not draw out the poisons. In these cases, something containing more sunlight than rainwater must be used, and that something is fruit-juice. The heat and drawing-power of fully-ripened fermenting apple-pulp is enormous; it will reduce varicose veins in about a week, and will draw the poisons from a diseased bone or tissue in a few weeks, if used persistently. All that is needed is a piece of clean linen, wrung out in rainwater, on one half of which the apple-pulp is spread. Having covered this with the other half of the linen, the poultice is applied to the affected area. It should be large enough to cover the area, and it can be warm, hot, or cold – the temperature does not matter, so long as it is the temperature most comfortable to the patient. The poultice must be changed every 3–4 hours, never allowing the area to get dry.

A method of treatment which has been used by the Chinese for thousands of years is called 'Acupuncture'. This also is designed to draw out poisons from the body and thus to encourage and promote self-healing.

225

It has recently been revived, and is used for conditions caused by toxaemia (impure bloodstream). It is also used for certain diseases of the central nervous system, for prolapsed intervertebral disc (commonly called slipped disc), and sometimes for acute appendicitis which it often cures without surgery.

In ancient times, before the human race lost its self-cleansing and self-restorative powers, an inflamed appendix would probably have terminated in a large abscess on the surface of the abdomen, as a result of hot rainwater (or apple-pulp) compresses over the painful area. Today, having forsaken natural living and natural foods, Man has lost the vitality to cure himself. This vitality is derived only from 'right eating, right living, and right thinking', and it will give him the strength either to cast out his own disease, or, if surgery is necessary, to make a rapid and complete recovery. For the greatest miracle of surgery is useless if the patient does not possess sufficient vitality to recover from it. That is why one often hears the remark, 'The operation was successful, but the patient died'.

In later times, during the eighteenth and nineteenth centuries, Malvern in Worcestershire became a popular health resort because of the curative power of its waters, which came from a well called the Holy Well and from St. Ann's springs. These waters were used with great success by Drs. Gully and Wilson who lived and practised in Malvern at that time, and who are reputed to have cured many sick and dying patients who flocked to Malvern from all over the world.

Chronic disease is a vicious circle out of which Man cannot extricate himself except by his own vitality, i.e. by his own innate recuperative powers which stem from his vitality. These powers are strengthened and increased by means of REST. This includes rest from noise and other distractions, from worries, etc., and possibly from solid food for short periods, now and then. A fleshless diet of natural compost-grown foods, eaten raw as far as possible, and a daily cleansing of the body, following a complete and thorough evacuation of the bowels, is also necessary for the building-up of vitality and of the natural ability to recuperate. *For, if the vitality – the life-force – can be raised sufficiently, all disease can be kept at bay or thrown off if it has developed.* Even cancer sufferers can take comfort from this fact. However, we should always bear in mind that 'life itself is an incurable disease' – that death is, sooner or later, inevitable, though it need not be sooner if due regard is paid to 'right eating, right living, and right thinking', and all that these three conditions entail.

In view of the fact that our atmosphere is polluted by so many poisonous substances nowadays, including 'fall-out' from atom bomb testings, it is probably safer to use distilled water for drinking than filtered rainwater, though filtered rainwater is best for washing in. To filter tapwater, an easily detached filter made by Safari Ltd. can be fitted to the kitchen tap (see page 9). The name of a firm that manufactures distilling-plant can be obtained from your local water company. Filters for filtering rainwater can be obtained from a big store such as Harrods in London.

British Spas

Name of Spa	Ailments Treated There
Bath	Gout and all forms of rheumatism and arthritis.
Bridge of Allen	Itching skin diseases.
Buxton	Gout, arthritis, and fibrositis.
Cheltenham	Gastro-intestinal catarrh, liver dysfunction, paralysis, muscular spasm (treated externally).
Droitwich (Brine Baths)	Arthritis (treated externally).
Harrogate	Liver dysfunction, constipation, obesity, diabetes.

Name of Spa	Ailments Treated There
Leamington Spa	Constipation, kidney and bladder troubles.
Llandrindrod Wells	Goutiness, gouty skin diseases, gouty-nephritis, cystitis.
Malvern (Holy Well)	Skin and eye troubles.
Trefriw Spa	Anaemia and all ailments due to shortage of iron.
Woodhall Spa	Naso-pharyngeal catarrh, laryngitis, etc.

Continental Spas

A guide to the spas of Germany, Czechoslovakia, and Bavaria can be obtained from the tourist office of these countries.

ZONE-THERAPY, AND YOUR FEET

The feet should be washed every day, then massaged for a few minutes, after drying with a rough towel, paying particular attention to any tender spots on the soles or sides of the feet or backs of the heels. These tender spots, if found, should be given deep friction with the tips of the fingers or thumb, till the tenderness vanishes. This is self-administered 'Zone-Therapy'. If there are no tender spots, then all is well with you, and all your internal parts are functioning normally; but if you find a tender spot, press and massage it until the tenderness disappears – or, better still, get a masseur to do it for you, not just once, but 2–3 times a week. Any painful spot (or zone) is an indication that something is amiss with the internal organ with which that particular zone is connected by longitudinal lines of force (meridians). Zone therapy is very similar to Acupuncture, the Chinese therapy first used by Chinese doctors over 5,000 years ago (and still used). It is the treatment of organic dysfunction by reflex action. (For further information, see 'Zone-Therapy' in

228

The Natural Home Physician by Eric Powell, N.D. (Health Science Press).)

A hot foot-bath with mustard in it is a good remedy not only for chills or a cold in the head but also for congestive headache. For sore and painful feet due to rheumatism or gout, the water should contain a good handful of common Epsom salts. For lumbago sufferers, the water should contain a tablespoonful of powdered flowers of sulphur, and some of the powder should be sprinkled into the feet of socks or stockings. For chilblains and poor circulation, the feet should be held for 3–4 minutes first in a hot bath, then for 1 minute in a cold one, repeating this process 4–5 times. Socks or stockings should be changed every day, as it is largely through the pores of the feet that the body gets rid of toxic wastes.

Corns and callouses can be softened by anointing them with oil of turps after each foot-bath. They will then be easily removable after a few days.

HOW TO BE HEALTHY ON A VEGETARIAN OR VEGAN DIET

Like most things, this is not difficult when you know how. In this instance, 'knowing how' means knowing which plant-foods take the place of animal-flesh, and how best to combine them to obtain as complete a protein-food as animal-flesh – for most of them are 'incomplete' proteins (i.e. proteins lacking one or more of the eight essential amino-acids that the body cannot manufacture itself), and, in order to convert them into 'complete' proteins, these incomplete proteins have to be combined with others which contain the amino-acids they lack. Moreover, this combining of their complementary amino-acids *must* take place at one and the same meal.

For example, if an incomplete protein such as soya beans,

which has a low content of one of the essential amino-acids called methionine, is eaten at, say, the midday meal, and another incomplete protein with a high content of methionine some hours later (or even only one hour later), the amino-acids that the beans *do* contain do not wait around for the missing methionine which the protein of the later meal contains, and then combine with it to form a 'complete' protein. This is not what happens – the time gap between the two meals prevents it. This means that no 'complete' protein, which is the only sort of any use for body-building, has been eaten that day. So the body suffers a protein deficiency which, if continued, will inevitably lead to ill-health – possibly, in time, to disease.

A 'complete' protein contains the eight essential amino-acids that the body cannot manufacture itself. These eight amino-acids are: Leucine, Isoleucine, Lysine, Methionine, Phenylalanine, Threonine, Tryptophan, and Valine. Given these eight essential ones, the body can, and does, manufacture the other fourteen. Eggs, cheese, milk, and yeast are 'complete' protein foods. Protein enters into the composition of so many body-components that its importance cannot be over-estimated. For instance, it is the chief ingredient of the red blood-cells, of the white blood-cells, of the gamma-globulins (better known as 'anti-bodies' which are part of the defence corps of the body), and of the many digestive enzymes. It is also the chief ingredient of 'hormones' (chemical messengers) and of albumin (a substance made by the liver from protein). This substance, circulating in the bloodstream, has the power to draw out of the tissues into the bloodstream the fluids which contain waste-products. These are then carried away by the bloodstream to the excretory organs.

A shortage of first-glass protein means that the liver is unable to make sufficient albumin, which means that the tissue-fluids (containing the waste-products) will not be drawn into the bloodstream and removed from the body. They will remain in the tissues, giving them an appearance of over-puffiness and swelling (e.g. round the ankles, wrists, and under the eyes). Indeed, in time, the whole body becomes waterlogged. People with such an appearance simply think that they are too fat, and they try to reduce their weight by cutting down their food-intake, including their protein-foods. This, of course, still further reduces the amount of protein available to the liver for the manufacture of albumin, the substance in the bloodstream which draws the fluids containing the waste-products out of the tissues into the bloodstream. The chubby appearance of children, which is usually associated with health, *can* be due to a retention of fluids and waste-products in the tissues. When a protein-rich diet is given to them, people soon lose their puffiness, and then often appear thin and underweight.

The secret of being a healthy vegetarian or vegan lies in knowing how to combine 'incomplete' (second class) protein-foods with others of the same kind, so as to obtain 'complete' (first class) protein-food – the only sort that is of any use to the body for the building of body-protein. To know how to do this a knowledge of the amino-acid content of the various vegetable-protein foods is required. This knowledge will enable you to combine them so that their amino-acids complement each other, and thus obtain a 'complete' protein-food from two or more 'incomplete' ones.

A simple alternative, which eliminates the need to acquire such knowledge, is always to eat some 'complete' protein food together with an incomplete one; incidentally, this will enhance the biological value of both sorts. But strict vegetarians (known as vegans) will not be willing to do this, because all the 'complete' protein-foods (except brewer's yeast) are animal products. This means that, unless vegans do acquire the necessary knowledge of how to combine 'incomplete' proteins so as to obtain a 'complete' protein-food, they will sooner or later suffer from protein deficiency, and this can lead to serious ill-health. Even if they do acquire the knowledge, they will probably suffer a vitamin B.12

deficiency, because vitamin B.12 is insufficiently supplied by a vegan diet. Vegans should, therefore, take the vitamin in tablet form, regularly and permanently. Most vegetarians do include animal-products (cheese, eggs, and milk) in their diet, so they will obtain small amounts of vitamin B.12 from these foods. Even so, it would be advisable for them also to take a vitamin B.12 tablet twice a week. (Vitamin B.12 is made from molds, not from any animal substance. Traces of it are obtained from wheatgerm, yeast, and soya-beans, but not sufficient.)

An egg is the perfect example of a 'complete' protein-food of high biological value, i.e. one that contains *all* the essential amino-acids in balanced proportions. The *quantity* of protein it contains is small compared with the quantity contained in the same weight of, say, peanuts, but the *quality* is high, because its protein contains all the essential amino-acids, whereas the protein of peanuts (like that of soya-beans) is low in methionine (one of the essential amino-acids).

Soya-beans and chick-peas come closest of all plant-foods to being 'complete' proteins, being low in methionine only. Next closest come peanuts and avocados. Peanuts are also low in methionine, but, by combining them with brazil nuts or sesame seeds, which have a high content of methionine, a 'complete' protein can be obtained. Likewise, natural whole cereals, such as wheat-grain (and bread made from it) have a low content of lysine (another of the essential amino-acids), but, by combining wheat and wheat-products with cashew nuts or soya, or chick-peas, all of which have a high lysine content, a 'complete' protein can be obtained. Thus it can be seen how 'incomplete' protein-foods can complement each other, and so produce a 'complete' protein-food. That is why it is wise to mix your incomplete protein-foods when planning a meal – or, as already suggested, to combine them with some 'complete' protein. (For further information on the subject, see *The Amino-acid Composition of Proteins and Foods* by Black and Bolling published in 1945 by Chas. C. Thomas.)

Many people eat several different kinds of 'complete' protein at a meal; for example, fish and meat and cheese, or fish and poultry and cheese, or fish and meat and milk. This is neither necessary nor advisable; it simply overtaxes the digestive organs, and the body derives no extra benefit therefrom. Just *one* 'complete' protein food is sufficient, at both a non-vegetarian meal *and* a vegetarian meal – though the biological value of the 'complete' protein can be enhanced by combining it with some 'incomplete' protein.

Foods such as eggs, cheese, milk, and brewer's yeast ('complete' proteins) supply *all* the essential amino-acids needed for the building of body-protein. Moreover, they supply them in the proportions in which they are found *in* body-protein. For example, if 100 grams of a protein food will replace 100 grams of body-protein, that food is said to be of the highest biological value; it has a biological value of 100%. Of the 'complete' proteins, milk proteins and egg proteins come nearest to such a high value, having a biological value of 56% and 62% respectively, and, when combined, they have a value approaching 100%. This is because their protein molecules are made up of a balanced proportion of all the essential amino-acids. They are therefore able to support body-building and body-maintenance.

A cereal such as wheat, which is low in lysine (one of the essential amino-acids), has a biological value of only 40%. To step-up this value, it should be combined with one of the foods that has a high biological value, such as milk, cheese, or eggs. Other vegetable-proteins of similar biological value, such as millet, rice, barley, sunflower seeds, sesame seeds, nuts, pulses, potatoes, avocados, etc., should likewise be combined and eaten with the high-value foods.

Milk, although not a perfect food because it does not contain all the minerals and vitamins required by the body, is nevertheless a 'complete' protein food. But, if it is to constitute the sole source of one's daily protein, a quart a day would have to be drunk. Therefore, except in illness (when it should be diluted with a little boiled water or soda-water), it is better to take it in small quantities, to supplement other foods that are not complete proteins, than as a sole source of one's protein.

Milk is a good source of calcium and of phosphorus, but is deficient in iron. It is a good source of vitamins A and K but has only a low content of the B group of vitamins, of vitamin C and of vitamin D. It is more easily absorbed than any other protein food when taken as part of a mixed diet in health, and as the sole article of diet in gastro-intestinal disorders. (In the latter case, it should be diluted with a little water or soda-water.) It has a far higher nutritive value than meat-extracts; moreover, it contains none of the harmful stimulants or prurines that they contain.

Skim milk (milk from which the fat has been extracted) is a concentrated high-protein food, an equally valuable source of 'complete' protein. So, too, is Casilan, a dried and powdered form of the casein of milk, which has a 90% protein content. Casilan is completely absorbed. It is invaluable in illness, being able to replace the need for all other protein-food and to neutralize over-acidity of the stomach.

The following table shows that 3 slices of wholewheat bread plus 1 pint of raw milk provides 30 grams of 'complete' protein. An adequately high-protein diet can, therefore, be obtained from a combination of milk, bread, cheese, eggs, and pulses, though the addition of watercress and of green leafy vegetables would further enhance its value – indeed, they are an essential part of any diet.

Wheat grains – in fact, all grains and beans, and seeds – double their value if they are 'sprouted'. This means first washing them thoroughly in warm water; then, after soaking them overnight, keeping them rinsed and moist in a warm place for a few days, at the end of which time they should be showing tiny green shoots. Allow these shoots to grow to about half an inch long, then nip them off and eat them in a mixed salad. 'Sprouting' grains and seeds doubles not only their protein content but also their vitamin, mineral, and enzyme content.

Table showing grams of protein in 100 grams (approx. 4 oz.
of the chief vegetarian-protein foods

('Complete' proteins in the following list have been marked*)

	grams
*Casilan (Dried Milk Protein)	90
Chick Peas	50
Soya Milk Powder	40
Soya Flour	43
*Brewer's Yeast (powder)	38
*Parmesan Cheese	36
Pine Kernels	31
*Cheddar Cheese	30
*Dutch Cheese	28
*Eggs (2)	28
Peanuts	28
Wheatgerm	26
Sunflower Seeds	25
St. Ivel (lactic acid) Cheese	23
Almonds	20
Sesame Seeds	18
Cashew Nuts	17
Buckwheat (Husked Grain)	15
Brazil Nuts	14
Oatmeal	14
Wholewheat Flour	13
Wholewheat Bread (3 rounds)	12
Millet Grain	12
Walnuts	12
Semolina	10
*Milk (Half a Pint)	9
Brown Barley (Whole Grain)	8
Lentils	7
Garden Peas	7
Pea Flour	7
Broad Beans	7
Brown Rice	3
Potatoes	2
Cabbage	2
Banana	1

It has been established that the average minimum daily protein requirement of an adult is $\frac{1}{2}$ gram for every kilogram (i.e. approx. 2 lb.) of body-weight. This means that a man weighing 70 kg. needs a minimum of 35 grams of protein daily, at least a third of which should be 'complete' (first class) protein; a 50/50 level would be even better and safer – safer because, as already stated, the body has to synthesize not only 14 amino-acids, red and white blood-cells, antibodies, enzymes, hormones, etc., but has also to synthesize 4 cell-nutrients – Inositol, Lipoic acid, Glutamine, and Coenzyme Q (and possibly others which have not yet been identified). All these can be synthesized only from the first class protein food eaten. It is thought that these (as yet) unidentified cell-nutrients (of whose existence there is evidence) are nutrients that protect the body from infectious diseases, just as self-produced cancer agents do. If they are underproduced, the body is more liable to disease of every sort.

It is essential that about half of one's daily intake of 'complete' protein-food should be eaten together with some carbohydrate (starch-containing) food, such as bread, potatoes, or cereals, etc. – otherwise it is useless for body-building and body-maintenance. The reason for this is that when the protein reaches the liver (having been broken down in the small intestines into its constituent amino-acids and then carried

Table showing relative amounts of the 8 essential amino-acids in the chief protein foods

FOOD	Iso-leucine	Leu-cine	Lysine	Methio-nine	Phenyl-alanine	Thre-onine	Trypt-ophan	Val-ine
			ANIMAL PROTEINS					
Casein (milk protein)	41	63	50	19	34	27	8	46
Cheese (Cheddar)	43	62	47	16	34	23	8	46
Cheese (Cottage)	37	68	53	17	34	30	6	36
Cheese (Cream)	37	65	51	16	39	29	5	38
Eggs	41	55	40	19	36	31	10	46
Milk (cow's)	40	62	49	*15*	30	29	9	43

FOOD	Iso-leucine	Leu-cine	Lysine	Methio-nine	Phenyl-alanine	Thre-onine	Trypt-ophan	Val-ine
			PLANT PROTEINS					
Barley (Brown)	25	40	*19*	8	30	19	7	29
Beans	35	53	46	*6*	34	27	5	38
Broccoli	24	31	28	9	22	23	7	32
Buckwheat Flour	23	36	36	11	23	24	7	32
Cabbage	18	25	29	6	13	17	5	19
Carrots	24	34	27	*5*	22	22	5	29
Cauliflower	27	42	35	12	19	26	8	37
Chick Peas	36	46	43	8	30	22	*5*	31
Cornmeal	29	81	*18*	11	28	25	*4*	32
Filberts	35	40	*17*	*6*	22	17	9	39
Lentils	33	44	38	*4*	27	22	5	34
Oats, and Oatmeal	30	44	*21*	8	31	19	7	35
Peanuts and peanut flour	25	38	22	*5*	31	*16*	6	31
Peas (cooked)	28	39	29	*5*	24	23	5	25
Peas (dried)	35	51	46	7	31	24	6	35
Pecan nuts	31	43	24	8	32	22	8	29
Peppers	23	24	26	8	28	26	4	17
Potatoes	27	31	33	8	27	24	6	33
Rice (brown)	28	51	*23*	10	30	23	6	41
Sesame seeds	26	46	*16*	17	40	19	9	24
Soybeans and *Soya-flour*	33	48	39	*8*	31	24	8	33
Soya-milk	29	51	45	*9*	33	29	8	31
Spinach	29	48	38	10	27	27	10	34
Sunflower seeds	29	40	20	*10*	28	21	8	31
Sweet potato	30	36	29	11	35	29	11	47
Tomatoes	18	25	26	4	18	21	5	17
Turnip tops	23	45	28	11	31	27	10	32
Wheat (whole-grain)	25	39	*16*	9	29	*15*	7	27
Wholewheat (flour)	25	39	*16*	9	29	*15*	7	27
Yeast (Brewer's)	32	43	44	11	25	32	9	37

to the liver by the bloodstream), its amino-acids are robbed of their nitrogen by powerful enzymes in the liver, and without its nitrogen it is useless for body-building. But, if carbohydrate food accompanies the protein food, the glucose derived from the break-down of the carbohydrate food curbs the activity of the enzymes which steal the nitrogen from the amino-acids.

An egg is a perfect example of protein that is biologically complete. Its amino-acid pattern should be referred to when wanting to compound a 'complete' protein from several 'incomplete' proteins. For example, the lysine content of wheat-protein is only 16 as compared with 40 which is the lysine content of the *same* weight of egg-protein. Its methionine content is also low as compared with the methionine content of the same weight of egg-protein.

Soya beans, sunflower seeds, and peanuts are low in methionine; sesame seeds are low in lysine but high in methionine, so they complement soya, sunflower seeds, and peanuts, converting the latter into 'complete' protein if eaten with them.

In the above list, plant foods (such as wheat) that have a low content of one (or more) of the essential amino-acids have had their low-content number printed in italics. Such foods should be eaten together with a food that has a higher content of that particular low-content amino-acid. The amino-acid content of an egg is a perfectly balanced one, and should serve as a perfect pattern for the compounding of a 'complete' protein from several 'incomplete' ones.

Table showing mineral content (in milligrams) in approx. 4 oz. of food

FOOD	Calcium	Phosphorus	Iron	Sodium	Potassium
Almond	234	504	4.7	4	773
Apricots (raw)	17	23	0.5	2	281
Apricots (dried and uncooked)	67	108	5.5	26	980
Asparagus (cooked)	21	50	0.6	1	183
Avocados (raw)	10	42	0.6	4	604
Bananas (raw)	8	26	0.7	1	370
Butter	20	16	0.0	987	23
Buttermilk	121	95	Trace	130	140
Barley (whole brown)	34	290	2.7	—	296
Beans (white cooked)	50	148	2.7	7	416
Beets (raw juiced)	16	33	0.7	60	335
Blackberries (raw)	32	19	0.9	1	170
Brazil nuts	186	693	3.4	1	715
Brussels Sprouts (cooked)	32	72	1.1	10	273
Buckwheat Flour	33	347	2.8	—	—
Cabbage (raw juiced)	49	29	0.4	20	233

FOOD	Calcium	Phosphorus	Iron	Sodium	Potassium
Cantaloupes (raw)	14	16	0.4	12	251
Carrots (raw)	37	36	0.7	47	341
Cashew nuts	38	373	3.8	15	464
Cauliflower (cooked)	21	42	0.7	9	206
Celery (raw)	39	28	0.3	126	341
Chick Peas (uncooked)	150	331	6.9	26	797
Cocoa	133	648	10.7	6	1,552
Coffee (dry powder)	179	383	5.6	72	3,256
Cucumbers (unpared)	25	27	1.1	6	160
Cheese (Cheddar)	750	478	1	700	82
Cheese (Cottage)	90	175	0.4	290	72
Cheese (Cream)	62	95	0.2	250	74
Cheese (Parmesan)	1,140	781	0.4	734	149
Dates	59	63	3	1	648
Eggs (cooked)	55	203	2.2	271	128
Figs	35	22	0.6	2	194
Hazel nuts	209	337	3.4	2	704
Horseradish	140	64	1.4	8	564
Kale (raw)	179	73	2.2	75	378
Lentils (cooked)	25	119	2.1	—	249
Milk (fresh)	117	92	Trace	50	140
Molasses	290	69	6	37	1,063
Onions (raw)	51	39	1	5	231
Onions (cooked)	24	29	4	7	110
Parsley	203	63	6.2	45	727
Peanuts	69	401	2.1	5	674
Peanut Flour	104	720	3.5	9	1,186
Peas (cooked)	56	76	0.5	—	119
Pecan nuts	73	289	2.4	—	603
Pistachio nuts	131	500	7.3	—	972
Potatoes (cooked in skins)	9	65	0.7	4	503
Pumpkin seeds	51	1,144	11.2	—	—
Radishes (raw)	30	31	1	18	322
Raisins (raw)	62	101	3.5	27	763
Rice (brown) (cooked)	12	73	0.5	282	70
Rye Flour	27	262	2.6	1	203
Sesame seeds	1,160	616	10.5	60	720
Soya Beans (cooked)	73	179	2.7	2	540
Soya flour	199	558	8.4	1	1,160
Soya milk powder	21	48	0.8	—	—
Spinach (cooked)	93	38	2.2	50	324
Sugar (brown)	85	19	3.4	30	344
Sunflower seeds	120	837	7.1	30	920
Syrup (maple)	104	8	1.2	10	176
Turnip tops	184	37	1.1	—	—
Walnuts	99	380	3.1	2	450
Wheat (whole)	7	52	0.5	212	48
Wholewheat flour	16	87	0.8	2	95
Wheatgerm	72	1,118	9.4	3	827
Yeast (Brewer's)	70–760	1,753	17.3	12	1,894
Yoghourt	112	87	—	47	132

Recommended daily intake of

Calcium,	Adults, 500–600 milligrams
	Growing children, 1 gram.
	Pregnant and nursing women, 1 gram.
Phosphorus,	Adults, 1.5 grams.
	Growing children, 1 gram.
Iron,	Adult men, 10 milligrams
	Adult women, 18 milligrams
	Growing children, 10–15 milligrams
	Pregnant women, 18 milligrams

There will be an adequate daily intake of potassium if brewer's yeast, soya products, peanuts, and molasses are eaten, and of sodium if wholewheat bread, cheese, butter, and fresh vegetables are eaten.

Chief sources of vitamins

VITAMIN A

Fish liver oils
Sheep's liver
Empire butter
Cheddar cheese
Dried whole milk
Fresh eggs
Kidney
Carrots
Parsley

Spinach
Turnip tops
Kale
Watercress
Dried apricots
Lettuce
Tomatoes
Prunes
Wheatgerm oil

VITAMIN B.1

Wheatgerm
Food yeast
Soya flour
Oatmeal
Dried peas
Liver
Cod's roe

Haricot beans
Peas
Dried milk
Wholewheat flour
Walnuts
Almonds
Peanuts

VITAMIN B.2
Milk

Butter

Egg-yolk

Liver

Food yeast

VITAMIN B.6
Brewer's yeast

VITAMIN B.12
Liver

Kidneys

Egg-yolk

Barmene

Alfalfa herb

B.12 Tablets (synthesized from molds)

VITAMIN C
Blackcurrants

Nasturtium leaves

Oranges

Lemons

Rose hips

Strawberries

Acerola

VITAMIN D
Fish liver oils

Sardines

Herrings

Mackerel

Salmon

Vitaminized margarine

Fresh eggs

Empire butter

VITAMIN E
All grains, seeds and nuts

Soya beans, soya-bean oil

Wheatgerm, wheatgerm oil

Royal jelly

In the above list, the sources with the highest content are italicized.

BANANAS – THEIR VALUE AS
FOOD AND MEDICINE

The food-value of bananas is fairly well known, but their medicinal usefulness and value is not generally realized or appreciated.

First, as a food, their protein includes 3 of the essential amino-acids, and they contain some vitamin A and vitamin C. They are an ideal food, especially for older people who often have chewing difficulties, being easy to chew, easy to digest, requiring no preparation, inexpensive, available all the year round, having a removable protective covering which prevents their edible portion from being contaminated by poison sprays and insecticides.

Bananas are low in sodium (one of the few protein foods that *are*), low in fats and cholesterol, rich in Essential-Fatty-Acids, in iron, and in natural fruit-sugar. Mashed up with a few spoonsful of soya-bean milk (Granogen) or plantmilk, they make a complete and highly nutritious meal. Needless to say, they should not be eaten in a half-ripe condition; but should be kept at room-temperature till they turn brown.

They are very suitable for people who are allergic to certain foods and who suffer in consequence from skin rashes, or digestive ailments, or asthma. Unlike other protein foods, many of which contain an amino-acid which these people cannot tolerate and which is the cause of their allergy, *bananas contain only benign amino-acids.*

Medicinally, they are of great value in a wide variety of ailments, including constipation *and* diarrhoea; this is due to the fact that they are normalizers of colonic functions. Their value in constipation is due to the fact that they are rich in pectin, which is a water-absorbent, and this gives them a bulk-producing ability. It is also due to their ability to change the bacteria in the intestines from the harmful putre-factive type of bacilli to the beneficial acidophyllus bacilli.

For colitis, ulcerative colitis, and spastic constipation, in all of which conditions irritating foods must be eliminated from the diet, yet where bulk is needed to ensure normal bowel movements, bananas are the ideal food, being bland, smooth, easily-digested, and slightly laxative.

For people with duodenal or gastric ulcer, they are also an ideal food. Bananas neutralize the over-acidity of the gastric juices, which is the cause of the ulceration, and they reduce irritation of the ulcer by coating the lining of the stomach.

Bananas are helpful in uraemia (a toxic condition of the blood due to kidney congestion and dysfunction). A diet of bananas only, for 3–4 days, eating 8–9 bananas a day and nothing else, is advised for people with kidney troubles (including nephritis, and gout).

Being low in sodium, fats, and cholesterol, they are a valuable food for people with heart troubles.

They are of great value also in coeliac disease (a children's disease), the symptoms of which are loss of appetite, dislike of food, persistent diarrhoea, intestinal pain, loss of weight, anaemia, and malnutrition. It has been found that the child will often vomit all foods other than bananas; these it seems to relish and to be able to digest.

Bananas are of great value to people who are on a reducing diet, and anxious to lose weight. They are low in calories, yet high in food-value. The diet of people with obesity or dropsy should contain no sodium-chloride (salt) and should consist of foods with a low sodium content. Bananas contain practically no sodium, hence their suitability for overweight people, as also for dropsical people. These people are unable to utilize the sodium in the foods they eat; the consequence is it accumulates in the tissues causing overweight because of its power of attracting fluids. Thus it is the liquid retained in the tissues, not the tissues themselves, that cause the overweight.

APPLE-CIDER VINEGAR

This deserves special mention, as it is a splendid and absolutely safe remedy for so many ailments. Here is a list of some of them: indigestion, due to a deficiency of gastric juices, because it closely resembles these juices; intestinal putrefaction, because it encourages the growth of beneficial bacteria in the intestines; calcium deficiency, because it helps the body to absorb the calcium it obtains from food; obesity, because this is often due to improper oxidation (burning-up) of food-stuffs, and cider-vinegar increases oxidation; over-frequent desire to pass water, because this is often caused by either an over-alkaline or an over-acid state of the urine, and cider-vinegar restores the alkaline-acid balance; high blood-pressure and difficult menstruation (both of which can be due to the blood being too thick) because cider-vinegar regulates the consistency of the blood, making it thinner and therefore freer-flowing; infections of the throat, nose, and larynx, because of its powerful germ-killing properties (even streptococcal germs); auto-intoxication (self-poisoning), because it detoxicates the poisons that accumulate in the liver and assists their expulsion from the body; constipation, because, for the complete elimination of all body-wastes from the bowel, a substance called pectin is necessary, and cider-vinegar contains pectin. So, too, do apples, and sunflower seeds. (Pectin has the power to attract water; this combines with the food-residues in the bowel and makes them swell, thus producing 'bulk', without which there can be no vigorous action of the bowels, and therefore no proper and complete elimination of waste-products); diarrhoea (unless due to some serious disorder), because diarrhoea is an effort made by the body to get rid of poisons, and cider-vinegar is an antiseptic which helps to remove the poisons.

Food-poisoning (suspected ptomaine poisoning). For this, put 1 teaspoonful of cider-vinegar into a glassful of cold water and sip 2 teaspoonfuls of the mixture every 5 minutes. Then less frequently as the pain and discomfort decrease.

There are many other ailments and disorders for which cider-vinegar can be used with great benefit. They are: ear, nose, eye, and throat troubles.

Ear discharge. For this, the sufferer takes one teaspoonful of the vinegar in a glassful of water, mid-morning and mid-afternoon. Biochemic remedies may also be necessary, to make good mineral deficiencies in the blood which are the underlying cause of the discharge. (See *The Biochemic Prescriber*, by Eric Powell, N.D., Health Science Press.)

Stuffy nose. This can be cleared by inhaling the steam given off from the cider-vinegar heated in a small pan.

Tired eyes. Vision can be greatly improved if 1 teaspoonful of cider-vinegar is taken in a glassful of water between meals, 2–3 times a day, for 1–2 months. A little honey makes the drink even more beneficial, because honey contains many minerals, including potassium and silica, a deficiency of which may be the underlying cause of the tiredness. Cider-vinegar with honey is also an excellent remedy for *cataract* (for the same reason).

Throat troubles. Sore throat, tickling cough, laryngitis, and pharyngitis, can all be relieved by gargling with cider-vinegar (1 teaspoonful in a glassful of warm water). Gargle with some of the mixture, then swallow a mouthful.

For the relief of Asthma, the dose should be 1 tablespoonful of the vinegar to a glassful of water, and the mixture should be sipped slowly, so that it takes $\frac{1}{2}$ hour to drink the whole glassful.

Post-operative haemorrhage and Haemophilia. Cidervinegar (1 teaspoonful in $\frac{1}{2}$ glassful of water) taken between meals 2–3 times a day for a month, before operations (or permanently in the case of haemophilia) will greatly reduce the risk of haemorrhage (for example, after excision of tonsils, adenoids, or polypi).

BOOKS FOR FURTHER READING

The Bach Flower Books, Dr. Edward Bach (The C. W. Daniel Co.)

Food is your best medicine, Dr. Bieler, M.D. (Neville Spearman)

Nature's Medicines, Richard Lucas (Neville Spearman)

Nutrition and Health, McCarrison and Sinclair (Faber & Faber)

Health via Food, Dr. Howard Hay (Harrap)

Nutrition against Disease, Dr. Roger Williams (Pitman, U.S.A.)

Superior Nutrition, Dr. Shelton (Brit. Natural Hygiene Society)

Food-combining made easy, Dr. Tilden (Brit. Natural Hygiene Society)

Food for the Golden Age, Frank Wilson (The C. W. Daniel Co.)

Food-reform Cook-book, Vivienne Quick (Gateway Book Co.)

Your Daily Bread, Doris Grant (Faber & Faber)

Housewives, Beware, Doris Grant (Faber & Faber)

Chemicals in Food, Dr. Franklin Bicknell (Faber & Faber)

The Blood-Poisoners. Lionel Dole (Gateway Book Co.)

The Master Key to Health, Dr. Rasmus Alsaker (Harrap)

Our Synthetic Environment, Lewis Herber (Jonathan Cape)

Our Daily Poison, Leonard Wickenden (Devin-Adair, New York)

Our Poisoned Earth & Sky, J. I. Rodale (Rodale Press)

The Living Soil, Lady Eve Balfour (Oxford University Press)

The Soil and Health, Sir Albert Howard (Oxford University Press)

The Earth's Green Carpet, Lady Howard (Rodale Press)

The Compost Gardener, F. C. King (T. Wilson & Son)

Nutritive Value in Crops, Professor Schuphan (Faber & Faber)

Soil, Grass, and Cancer, Andre Voisin (Crosby Lockwood)

The Stuff Man's Made Of, Jorian Jenks (Faber & Faber)

The Prevention of Incurable Disease, Dr. Bircher-Benner (James Clarke)

The Curability of Cancer, Dr. P. Kersch (Brit. Biochemic Assocn.)

Victory over Cancer, Cyril Scott (Gateway Book Co.)

Cancer, its Genesis and Treatment, Dr. Forbes-Ross (Methuen & Co.)

Cancer, its Dietetic Cause and Cure, Dr. Maud Fere (Gateway Book Co.)

Cancer, its Cause and Prevention, J. Ellis Barker (Health Science Press)

Everybody's Guide to Nature Cure, Harry Benjamin (Gateway Book Co.)

Eat Nature's Food and Live Long, Dr. Josiah Oldfield (The C. W. Daniel Co.)

Children's Health and Happiness, Margaret Brady, M.SC (Gateway Book Co.)

The Natural Home Physician, Eric Powell, N.D. (Health Science Press)

Foods for Good Health and Healing, Dr. Dulley Wright (Health Science Press)

Building a Healthy Heart, Eric Powell, N.D. (Health Science Press)

Your Key to a Healthy Heart, Herbert Bailey (Chilton Books)

The Herbal Cure of Duodenal Ulcers and Gallstones, Capt. Frank Roberts, M.N.I.M.H. (The Herbal Dispensaries, Hanham, Nr. Bristol)

Encyclopaedia of Digestive Disorders, Capt. Frank Roberts, M.N.I.M.H. (Thorsons Ltd.)

Books for Further Reading

Fruit Dishes & Raw Vegetables, Dr. Bircher-Benner (The C. W. Daniel Co.)

Children's Diet, Dr. Bircher-Benner (The C. W. Daniel Co.)

Get Well Naturally, Linda Clarke (Devin-Adair Co., New York)

Herbal Remedies & Recipes, Mary Thorne-Quelch (Faber & Faber)

Let's Eat Right to Keep Fit, Adelle Davis (Devin-Adair Co., New York)

Your Heart and Vitamin E, E. & W. Shute (Devin-Adair Co., New York)

You can Add Years to Your Heart, P. E. Norris (Thorsons Ltd.)

The Raw-Food Treatment of Cancer & Other Diseases, Dr. Kirstin Nolfi (The Vegetarian Society)

The Seven Keys to Colour Healing, Roland Hunt (The C. W. Daniel Co.)

Homoeopathy for the First-Aider, Dr. Dorothy Shepherd (Health Science Press)

Why Kill for Food, Geoffrey Rudd (The Vegetarian Society)

Healing by Water, T. Hartley-Hennessy (The C. W. Daniel Co.)

Diet in Sinus Infections, Dr. E. V. Ullmann (Macmillan & Co.)

Biotonic Therapy, Maryla de Chrapowicki (The C. W. Daniel Co.)

Some Adventures in Healing, Dr. Graupner (Gollancz)

Cosmos, Man and Society, Dr. Szekery (The C. W. Daniel Co.)

Medicine Tomorrow, Dr. Szekery (The C. W. Daniel Co.)

The Nature Doctor, Dr. Vogel (Swiss Health Products)

Acknowledgements

The author is indebted to the following book for various extracts: *Metabolism* published by The Federation of American Societies for Experimental Biology.

248

INDEX

Acid dyspepsia, 41; remedy for, 41–2

Acidophillus bacilli, 200

Acne, 42; treatment, 42; diet, 42–3

A.C.T.H., 52; use of in treatment of arthritis, 52

Acupuncture, 50, 156, 225, 228

Acute illness, symptoms of, 17

Adenoids and tonsils (enlarged), 43; treatment of, 44–5

Aluminium cooking vessels, dangers in use of, 14

Amino acids, 229, 232, 236, 237, 242

Anabolism, 7

Anaemia, 45; causes of, 45, 48; treatment, 45; remedying acids-deficiency, 45–6; pernicious, 47; cause and remedy, 47–8

Angina pectoris, 48; relieving of, 48–9

Anthrone Test, 215

Appendicitis, 49; nature-cure treatment of, 49–50

Apple-cider vinegar, 244–6; as remedy for many ailments, 244–6

Arnica tincture, 34

Arteriosclerosis, 50; causes of, 50–1

Arthritis, 51–5; causes of, 51–2; treatment, 54; biochemic remedies, 55; homoeopathic remedy, 55

Asthma, 55–8; causes of, 55–6; diet reform as help in, 56–7; remedies, 57–8; beneficial use of shower baths for, 57; cardiac, 58; treatment of, 58

Auto-immunity, 87

Bach, Dr. Edward, 211; thirty-eight flower remedies of, 211

Backwardness in children, 59

Bacteria, 200

Baldness, 59; treatment for, 59

Banana, value of as food and medicine, 242–3

Barker, J. Ellis, 77; views on surgery to cure cancer, 77

Bean-pod soup, 198; as remedy for sundry ailments, 198

Beard, Dr. Howard, 80, 214; view on cancer, 214–17; Works, *A New Approach to the Conquest of Cancer*, 214q.

Belladonna, 35

Bilious attack, 59–60; homoeopathic remedy for, 60

Biochemic remedies, 26–7

Bircher-Benner Clinic, 222

Blackheads, suppurating, treatment of, 43

Bladder, stone in, 62; homoeopathic remedy, 62; liquid remedies, 62–3

Bladder and kidney troubles, 60–3; diet as aid in, 60–1; homoeopathic remedy, 61

Blistering, 24

Blond, Kasper, 67; theory of cause of cancer, 68

Blood-letting (Venesection), 23

Blood-purifiers, 63–4; 'macro-biotic' diet, 64

Index

Body: functioning of, 7; factors in resistance of body to disease, 15–16
Body cleansing, 16
Boils and carbuncles, 64–5; drawing 64
Bowel purging, 16
Brain-fag, 65
Bright's Disease, 65; remedy for, 65
British spas, list of, 227–8
Bronchial catarrh, 66; remedy for, 66
Bronchitis and Broncho-pneumonia, 66; cure for, 66; acute, remedy for, 84; chronic, remedy for, 84
Bunions, 66; to relieve, 66

Calendula tincture, 33
Camomile tea, 199; use of, 199
Camphorated oil, 35, 66
Carey, Dr. George, 27; Works, *The Biochemic System of Medicine*, 27q.
Cancer, 67–80; cause of, 67–70, 75–6; prevention of, 70, 76; of breast and/or lung, 79; of rectum, 79; of lymph glands, spleen and liver, 80; of skin, 80; of blood (Leukaemia), 80; anti-tumour remedies, 80; use of Podophyllin in skin cancer, 180; insulin treatment for, 218
Castor oil, 36
Catalase, 70–1, 75
Catarrh, 80–5; importance of correct feeding in, 81; quickest way to rid, 81–2; natural remedies for, 83
Catarrh, nasal (chronic), 83–4; medical treatment of, 83; biochemic remedy for, 83; herbal remedy for, 83–4
Catarrh, bronchial, 84; homoeo-pathic remedy for, 84; of eustachian tubes, remedy for, 84; of stomach, remedies for, 84–5; of vagina (Leucorrhea), remedy for, 85

Cell-metabolism, 7–8
Cell-nutrients, 236
Cell-respiration, 8, 19; rate of, 8
Cell-structure, 8
Change of life, 86
Chapped hands, 85
Chest complaints, treatment of, 86
Chilblains, 85; remedy for, 85
Childbirth (painless), 86
Children's ailments, 86–7; teething troubles, remedy for, 86
Chymotrypsin, 80, 214–15, 216
Cider-vinegar, 36
Cinnamon, 35
Circulatory disturbances, 87–8; treatment of, 87–8
Clark, Linda, 12, 153; Works, *Get Well Naturally*, 12q., 153q.
Claydos, 188
Coeliac disease, 88–9; diet for, 88–9
Co-enzyme Q, 236
Colchicine, 80
Cold, common, 89–91; treatment of, 89–91
Coli Communis bacilli, 200
Colitis, 91–2; kinds of, 91; treatment of, 91–2; diet correction in, 92; ulcerative, 93–5; diet for, 94–5
Comfrey tea, 198–9; use of, 198–9
Composition powder, 35
Compton-Burnett, Dr., 45
Constipation, 95–100; cause of, 95–7; treatment of, 98–100
Cooking vegetables, correct method of, 12
Corns and callouses, 100; treatment of, 229

250